Inventing the NIH

Victoria A. Harden

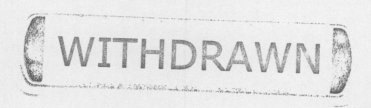

Inventing the NIH

*Federal Biomedical
Research Policy,
1887–1937*

The Johns Hopkins University Press
Baltimore and London

The opinions and conclusions expressed in this book are entirely those of the author and not of the National Institutes of Health.

The Johns Hopkins University Press, 701 West 40th Street, Baltimore, Maryland 21211
The Johns Hopkins Press Ltd., London

The paper used in this publication meets the minimum requirements of American National Standard for Information Sciences—Permanence of Paper for Printed Library Materials, ANSI Z39.48-1984.

Library of Congress Cataloging-in-Publication Data

Harden, Victoria A.
   Inventing the NIH.

   Bibliography: p.
   Includes index.
   1. National Institutes of Health (U.S.)—History. 2. Medicine—Research—Government policy—United States—History. 3. Public health—Research—Government policy—United States—History. 4. Federal aid to medical research—United States—History. I. Title.
RA11.D6H37 1986   353.0084   85-24070
ISBN 0-8018-3071-0 (alk. paper)

To Bob, Durward, and Emily

Contents

Illustrations

Preface

In this book I have attempted to elucidate the origins and early history of the National Institutes of Health (NIH), from their beginning as a one room bacteriological laboratory in 1887 through the first seven years, from 1930 through 1937, of operation as the National Institute of Health. It is surprising how little has been written about the early history of federal biomedical research in the United States, and one volume cannot do justice to all aspects of its development. This study focuses on factors that affected the development of a federal biomedical research policy, particularly changing social attitudes, economic pressures, the professionalization of science and public health, and occasionally even the results of research undertaken by federal scientists.

Throughout the years of research for this book, I have found a lively interest in the history of this country's foremost medical research facility. I am grateful to the many people who offered encouragement, information, and suggestions for new sources. Many of them are named in the Note on Sources, but it is impossible to list everyone.

The initial portion of the research for this book, which grew out of my doctoral dissertation at Emory University, was done in 1980 while I held an Emory graduate fellowship. Additional research and writing were done from 1981 through 1984. For the academic year 1981–1982 I held a predoctoral fellowship in the Medical Sciences Division, the National Museum of American History, the Smithsonian Institution, and a simultaneous grant awarded by the National Library of Medicine (LM 03782). That grant was extended for an additional year. I spent the 1983–1984 academic year as a postdoctoral fellow at the Institute of the History of Medicine of the Johns Hopkins University

Medical School, also under the auspices of a National Library of Medicine grant (LM 04093). I wish to acknowledge with gratitude the generous support of these institutions.

Historians would find their work much more difficult, if not impossible, without the help of librarians and archivists. For this book I have incurred debts to many, a number of whom I have acknowledged in the Note on Sources. Special thanks must go to Linda Matthews and her associates in the Special Collections Department, Robert W. Woodruff Library, Emory University; to the library staff at the National Museum of American History of the Smithsonian Institution; and to Doris Thibodeau in the Institute of the History of Medicine, Welch Library, the Johns Hopkins University Medical School.

The assistance of other individuals also proved especially valuable. Wyndham Miles, historian at the National Library of Medicine, encouraged my efforts from the beginning and shared with me many important sources he had collected over the years. Germaine Reed, professor of history at the Georgia Institute of Technology, kindly provided me with information from her research for a biography of Charles Holmes Herty. Conversations with John Parascandola, chief of the Division of the History of Medicine at the National Library of Medicine, who was working on a cognate theme while still on the faculty at the University of Wisconsin, proved stimulating to my research. Owsei Temkin, professor emeritus at the Institute of the History of Medicine, the Johns Hopkins University Medical School, provided encouragement and wise advice at a crucial time. A number of administrators at the National Institutes of Health, who are named in the Note on Sources, read and offered helpful suggestions on the Epilogue. Special thanks for assistance on this portion of the book is due NIH Director James B. Wyngaarden and his immediate predecessor, Donald S. Fredrickson. My son, C. Durward McDonell III, typed the manuscript for the book on a word processor with precision, patience, and good humor.

Most especially I wish to thank Professor James Harvey Young, now emeritus, at Emory University. He served as my dissertation advisor and has continued to offer advice, criticism, and moral support for my efforts. Professor Young patiently read and edited, to good advantage, more versions of this manuscript, as it has progressed from a seminar paper to book form, than he probably cares to remember. The debt of gratitude I owe to him can never be fully repaid.

Producing any work of this size is, of course, a family affair. My son, in addition to typing the manuscript, introduced me to the family of John W. Kerr, whose manuscripts were subsequently made available for this study. My daughter, Emily V. McDonell, has lived a good part of her life thinking of this book as practically another member of the family. My husband, Robert L. Berger, has been my partner and mainstay in this undertaking. His critical reading of the manuscript, moral support, and enormous energy have both benefited this book and sustained its author.

INTRODUCTION:
Inventing the NIH

If we did not have NIH we would have to invent it.
Robert M. Bock, 1980

The focal point for health research in the United States in the 1980s is the National Institutes of Health (NIH), the federal government's principal biomedical research agency. The eleven component institutes employ over fourteen thousand physicians, scientists, and support staff, most of whom work on a 317-acre campus in Bethesda, Maryland. The Institutes provide over 30 percent of all money allotted for the support of health research and development in the United States and nearly 70 percent of the total federal funds expended for support of medical research in universities.[1]

The Institutes concern themselves with fundamental, or basic, research, the application of which to medical problems cannot readily be demonstrated, and with applied research such as experimental chemotherapy for cancer or large-scale clinical trials of new drugs. Since the late 1960s budgetary constraints have generated debate over the allocation of scarce funds between the two types of research.[2] This debate generally recognizes the inherent interrelatedness of basic and applied research and therefore is primarily concerned with emphasizing one or the other, not abandoning either. Almost no one has questioned the assumption that federal support of basic as well as applied biomedical research is a proper function of the federal government. The *Washington Post,* for example, in a 1982 editorial on the federal science budget, stated: "Basic research, a long-range investment for the benefit of all society, is properly and necessarily the responsibility of the federal government."[3] Similarly, most members of the biomedical community support the concept of government patronage for research. Robert M. Bock, chairman of the Public Affairs

Committee of the Federation of American Societies for Experimental Biology, remarked in 1980: "If we did not have NIH we would have to invent it. Someone has written and many believe, that NIH is one of the truly remarkable social inventions of the ages."[4]

Bock was correct in describing the National Institutes of Health as an "invention," because the kinds of problems studied by the Institutes, the practice of maintaining both an intramural staff of researchers and an extramural program that funds other projects across the United States, and the very questions that in the late twentieth century are at the center of controversy are all the product of nearly one hundred years of inventive policy making by public health leaders, by scientists, by the Public Health Service bureaucracy, and by the United States Congress. The mushrooming growth that has occurred in this federal biomedical research agency since World War II has overshadowed its institutional roots, yet this very expansion occurred within the context of a heritage from both the public health and the scientific research communities, a legacy that continues to be significant in shaping policy. The purpose of this book is to elucidate the origins of the Institutes in these two communities and to examine the ways in which members of these groups interacted in the political arena to develop a federal biomedical research policy before 1937, the year in which the National Cancer Institute was created and the later expansion of NIH effectively launched.

The broad consensus in favor of government-supported biomedical research that has characterized the second half of the twentieth century is a relatively recent phenomenon in American history. The United States Constitution provided no specific mechanism for the support of either science or medicine beyond patent protection and the regulation of interstate commerce.[5] Throughout most of the nineteenth century, medical research was conducted by a few interested practicing physicians in their spare time. Even with the advent of the germ theory of disease and the concomitant possibility that the science of bacteriology could provide therapies for or preventive inoculations against infectious maladies, neither the people of the United States nor their elected representatives felt that it was proper for the federal government to support on a large scale institutions that would pursue such ends.

In 1887 the federal government did establish a laboratory of hygiene in its Marine Hospital Service. This was a bacteriological laboratory that assisted the Service in the diagnosis of infectious diseases among immigrants and performed other types of bacteriological work for Congress, the District of Columbia, and some states. Throughout the late nineteenth century, the Hygienic Laboratory, as it came to be called, conducted practical research such as analyzing the bacterial count in water wells, and, with the advent of Progressive Era regulatory legislation in the early twentieth century, enlarged its scope to include the enforcement of the Biologics Control Act of 1902.

The fortunes of this laboratory were tied in these early years to an ongoing debate between some public health leaders, who came to think of themselves as members of a "national health movement" because of their desire to centralize public health work in a national department of health, and the leaders of the Marine Hospital Service, who wished to see their agency develop into such a body. Ever attendant upon this debate were other voices in American society that vociferously opposed the efforts of both of these other groups. Because of the Laboratory's status as one aspect of a broader public health effort, there was no effort made to advance research as a separate concern from this larger issue.

Similar endeavors to centralize other scientific disciplines were made in the late nineteenth century. A. Hunter Dupree has analyzed these movements and the opposition to them, and has observed that science of all types is a "profoundly plural" undertaking in the United States.[6] One reason for the failure of such proposals was the deeply ingrained American opposition to the establishment of government patronage for any special group.[7] Among members of the scientific research community, moreover, government funding implied the specter of government control over research priorities. As late as 1928, for example, the noted chemist Atherton Seidell observed: "We [Americans] naturally question governmental participation in scientific matters because we feel that anything having a political flavor cannot be above suspicion."[8]

Yet by the 1920s scientific research, including medical research, had assumed a place of importance in the federal establishment and was beginning to include some basic researchers alongside the applied scientists who worked for agencies such as the Department of Agriculture or the Hygienic Laboratory. Progressive Era reforms such as the 1906 Pure Food and Drugs Act, enforced by the Department of Agriculture, had required that the government employ additional scientific experts to enforce the law. In this capacity, the scientist as bureaucrat became an accepted, valued part of the executive branch of government. During World War I, moreover, a large number of scientists worked for the government to solve many technological problems, especially those relating to chemical warfare. The experiences of chemists and other scientists as employees of the government called into question many of their traditional assumptions about government-sponsored research at the same time that the status of science and scientific medicine was increasing in the eyes of the public. Such a combination of changing perceptions opened the way in the second half of the 1920s to a reconsideration of the federal role in health research.

The transformation in medical research policy, which began in the Progressive Era and gathered momentum between 1918 and 1930, was not so dramatic as the sudden acceleration that followed World War II. I will argue, however, that what appeared as a sudden change in government policy after World War II was instead a "take-off" period, to borrow a phrase from W. W. Rostow's theory of take-off into economic growth, after a longer and less dramatic period of re-alignment, during which both the American people and the scientific research community came to support the concept of enlarged federal patronage for biomedical research. George Rosen termed such pre-liminary periods "critical periods" because it is during such times that underlying attitudes, in the case of policy shifts, are changed.[9]

In the following pages I hope to show how developments in the public health and scientific research communities contributed to the "invention" of what was known between 1930 and 1948 as the National Institute of Health. In the latter year, the creation of new institutes caused the name to be made plural. At the outset I should state that references to "communities" of biomedical scientists, public health leaders, and the like are used primarily for convenience and with no intent to convey the notion that members of any group were monolithic in their attitudes. Further, the very central words *medical research* and *biomedical science* are used to mean attempts to understand natural phenomena relating to the human body in states of health and disease, by specially trained people who are recognized by their colleagues generally through publications relating to their research efforts and through credentials awarded by universities. No attempt is made in this book to employ a class analysis approach to the events described. My aim is to elucidate the factors that contributed to the development of a National Institute of Health in the United States and to explain these developments as a part of the larger culture and the increasing federalization of all the sciences in the twentieth century.

The book is divided into three parts. Part One focuses on the origins of the Hygienic Laboratory in the context of the public health move-ment in the late nineteenth century. It also describes the development of the Laboratory to the mid-1920s as this occurred within the ongoing conflict between the national health movement and the Public Health Service. It concludes with the establishment of an alliance between these two groups, and analyzes proposed legislation that resulted from this agreement, legislation that provided for a modest expansion of the Laboratory. Part Two of the book traces the origins of an idea for a large national biomedical research institute to the experiences of chemists who worked with the Chemical Warfare Service during World War I, and who, after the war, proposed the creation of a privately funded chemotherapeutic research institute. It examines the reasons that the group was unable to find private-sector funding for the proposed institute and explains how the idea for such an institute inspired Louisiana senator Joseph Eugene Ransdell to introduce a bill for federal sponsorship of a similar facility that he chose to call the National Institute of Health. In Part Three of the book, the legislative histories of the two bills emerging from the public health and scientific research communities are traced within the context of the conservative political climate of the 1920s. The interactions of the proponents of each bill, sometimes competitive, sometimes supportive, are analyzed, as are the compromises to which each group agreed in order to win congressional approval. The final chapter of this section looks at the product of their handiwork—the newly created National Institute of Health. It examines bureaucratic policy making that occurred within the limitations of the Great Depression in the first seven years of the Institute's existence. The book concludes by surveying briefly the development of the mature Institutes in light of their historical antecedents.

PART ONE

Origins in Public Health

ONE
A Laboratory of Hygiene

In August, 1887, a bacteriological laboratory was established at the
port of New York.
*Annual Report of the Supervising Surgeon
of the Marine Hospital Service, 1888*

The National Institutes of Health trace their origin to a one
room bacteriological laboratory established in August 1887
in the Marine Hospital on Staten Island, New York. It is
not surprising that the United States government should
have spent "several hundred dollars" outfitting a laboratory at this
time, because the 1880s were a heroic decade of bacteriological discovery.[1] In 1882 the German physician Robert Koch had set forth his
postulates for definite identification of a particular bacterium as the
cause of a particular disease and demonstrated the tubercle bacillus
as the cause of tuberculosis. After this date the germ theory of disease,
which had previously been largely ignored by American physicians,
was rapidly accepted, at least by the leaders of the medical profession
in the United States.[2] Many of them traveled to Europe to study the
methods of bacteriology with Koch, French chemist Louis Pasteur,
or their associates.

In Europe this explosion of knowledge was the culmination of a
century of research in universities, and several leading European researchers were rewarded by their governments or by private subscriptions with laboratories in which further investigations could be
conducted.[3] No such research tradition had been established in the
United States; hence, American physicians and scientists sought to
incorporate the new knowledge and techniques in the emerging graduate programs in universities and in the few public health agencies
that had been formed since the Civil War. In 1887, the same year
that the federal laboratory was created, the Lawrence Experiment
Station was established in Massachusetts; the hygienic laboratory in
Ann Arbor, Michigan, was set up during the winter of 1887–88; and

the first municipal public health laboratory was founded in 1888 in Providence, Rhode Island.[4] Like its state and municipal counterparts, the federal government's laboratory was designated a "laboratory of hygiene," since bacteriological methods were employed primarily to serve the principal weapons of public health against disease at this time, sanitation and quarantine. As the years passed, this descriptive name gradually and without apparent design became transformed into the proper noun Hygienic Laboratory.

The establishment of the Hygienic Laboratory was not simply a practical decision to bring the latest šcientific methods to the work of sanitation. This laboratory was born amidst larger political debate over the need for and the organization of federal activity in health matters. Because of the rudimentary state of medical knowledge in the eighteenth century, the framers of the United States Constitution had not mentioned health as an area in which the federal government would be involved. From that time through the early nineteenth century, illness was considered a private affair, and when epidemic disease struck communities, civic leaders organized temporary committees to deal with the emergency.[5] After the Civil War a few of these bodies became permanent parts of municipal government. The federal government had established in 1798 a Marine Hospital Service for the purpose of providing medical care to merchant seamen. This Service, however, was composed of a decentralized chain of hospitals, funded by monthly deductions from the wages of the seamen and managed by one clerk in the Treasury Department who kept records of the accounts.[6] It was in no way a national federal public health agency.

In the middle of the nineteenth century, this situation began to change when European immigrants swelled the eastern seaboard cities of the United States. The slum conditions in which many of the immigrants lived contributed to epidemics and crime that had an impact on the entire community. Although the concept of microbial disease causation had not yet taken hold, the connection between squalid conditions and epidemics generated an interest in sanitation and quarantine as preventive measures, especially after John C. Griscom and Lemuel Shattuck published reports on the sanitary conditions in New York and Boston in 1845 and 1850, respectively.[7]

The sanitary and medical activities of the Civil War, furthermore, brought to prominence a number of physicians who wished to advance what was often called "sanitary science" in the United States. One of the most notable of these was John Shaw Billings of the United States Army.[8] Architect of the Johns Hopkins University Hospital, friend of Robert Koch, compiler of the *Index-Catalogue* of the library of the

Surgeon General of the Army, and initiator of *Index Medicus*, Billings was actively involved in many endeavors to promote public health and scientific medicine throughout the last decades of the nineteenth century. Shortly after the Civil War he made a survey of the existing Marine Hospitals and suggested to his friends in the administration of Ulysses S. Grant that the Marine Hospital Service would run more efficiently if it were reorganized under a central Supervising Surgeon based in Washington, D.C. A bill to this effect won congressional approval with the stipulation that the Supervising Surgeon must come from civilian life, a provision that blocked Billings's expected appointment to the post.[9] The person chosen in April 1871 to head the reorganized Service was John Maynard Woodworth, a former Army officer who had won acclaim as the physician who cared for Union casualties during General William Tecumseh Sherman's march through Georgia.[10] Thus rebuffed by Congress, the ambitious Billings turned his energies to supporting a movement for the establishment of a full-scale national department of health in the federal government, hoping to play a prominent role in its administration.

The idea of establishing a cabinet-level department of health was one of several goals shared by members of the American Public Health Association (APHA), an organization formed in 1872, just after the Marine Hospital Service had been reorganized. At the first annual meeting of the association in 1873, one speaker called for the creation of a "National Sanitary Bureau" in the federal government to promote knowledge of the most recent advances in sanitary science.[11] The idea was not unique to the APHA; in 1875 Henry I. Bowditch also outlined such a plan to the members of the American Medical Association at their annual meeting.[12] The arguments for a national department of health centered around the need for adequate administrative machinery to coordinate public health programs. Federal leadership was required, proponents said, because boards of health were rare and often underfunded on the state and local level, and, in any case, many problems transcended state boundaries.

Both Billings and Woodworth were active in the American Public Health Association, and each hoped to lead such a department. Billings proposed the establishment of a separate agency in the Interior Department; Woodworth argued for the expansion of the Marine Hospital Service into the public health arena. Their personal rivalry sparked a struggle that lasted over fifty years between the Service and public health leaders who desired a separate national department of health. To the development of medical research in the Hygienic Laboratory this contest was of the utmost importance. It helped to foster the establishment of the Laboratory, and throughout the next half century was one of the principal factors in the development of policy regarding the federal medical research effort.

The first campaign in the crusade was won by Billings. After the devastating yellow fever epidemic in the Mississippi Valley in 1878, Billings and others supporting the concept of a national health department convinced Congress to establish a National Board of Health.[13] With Billings as vice-president, the board made research grants to university faculty members who were interested in studying yellow fever, the first governmental grants ever awarded for medical research. The board was also assigned quarantine duties previously exercised by the Marine Hospital Service. Members of the board had some difficulties dealing with the representatives of several southern states over the quarantine issue, and the Marine Hospital Service worked actively to exploit the problems in order to regain its lost authority in this area. Exacerbating the situation was the sudden death of Supervising Surgeon Woodworth eleven days after the board's enabling legislation was enacted. The cause of Woodworth's death was not recorded, but one medical journal attributed it to overwork, and his successor as Supervising Surgeon, John B. Hamilton, stated that "persecution" from the proponents of the Board had been the cause.[14] The appropriation for the National Board of Health expired in 1883; under pressure from the Marine Hospital Service, it was not renewed. In 1893 the act establishing the Board was repealed.

Faced in the mid-1880s with an organization in name only, Billings sought to maintain his position through the establishment of another, permanent bureau. One of his strongest arguments to the House of Representatives Commerce Committee hearing the proposal in 1888 was that the proposed bureau would conduct "continuous scientific investigations" for the good of the public health. To counter Billings's argument, Supervising Surgeon Hamilton announced to the committee that the Marine Hospital Service was already conducting scientific investigations and disclosed the existence of the Hygienic Laboratory.[15] This revelation effectively stopped the creation of Billings's proposed bureau of health. The establishment of the Laboratory was announced formally in the Service's 1888 annual report, which stated simply: "In August, 1887, a bacteriological laboratory was established at the port of New York."[16]

The creation of the laboratory of hygiene was doubtless more, however, than a political stick with which the Marine Hospital Service could beat its opposition. Supervising Surgeon Woodworth had followed the bacteriological work of European investigators in the 1870s and had spent a year in the hospitals of Berlin and Vienna studying laboratory methods.[17] Walter Wyman, the Service officer in charge of the Marine Hospital at the port of New York, had also studied European laboratory techniques.[18] Granted power in 1883 to quarantine foreign ships entering United States ports if they harbored infectious diseases among their passengers, the Service had need of such assistance as bacteriological methods offered. It required only a qualified person who was free to assume the task of performing bacteriological work.

In 1886 a young physician joined the Service who had taken his medical degree at the Bellevue Hospital Medical College of New York University and had done postdoctoral work with Robert Koch in Germany and with Elie Metchnikoff at the Pasteur Institute in Paris.[19] Joseph James Kinyoun was sent to Wyman at the Staten Island Marine Hospital and given the authority to set up the laboratory of hygiene in "one of the rooms of the main hospital building, which had formerly done service as a museum for the 'Seamen's Fund and Retreat Hospital.' "[20] Kinyoun's Laboratory was equipped with pieces of scientific apparatus "modeled after those used in the laboratory of Dr. Koch" and was "supplied with Zeiss's latest improved microscope objectives and micro-photographic apparatus."[21] Animals were available for experimental purposes.

Kinyoun's first investigation was an "analysis of the waters of the New York Bay" to determine their power to sustain the life of the cholera spirillum.[22] This work and the subsequent identification of the cholera "comma bacillus" in the stools of immigrants represented the first bacteriological diagnosis of cholera in the Western Hemisphere.[23] Cholera and yellow fever were two of the most dreaded epidemic diseases at this time; they were logically the first problems to be attacked by the new Laboratory. And, indeed, a special investigation for the Louisiana board of health, consisting of experimental studies on the "supposed micro-organisms of yellow fever," was also conducted during the Laboratory's first year.[24]

These early studies were expanded to cover other problems found in merchant seamen and in immigrants, a second group for whom the Service was given greater responsibility in 1890.[25] Tuberculosis, typhoid fever, pneumonia, anthrax, malaria, and suppuration came under the scrutiny of the Hygienic Laboratory. Disinfection was also a major concern, and Kinyoun experimented with a variety of gases before settling on sulphur dioxide and formaldehyde as the disinfecting agents of choice.

In these early years Kinyoun did most of the laboratory work himself, aided from time to time by other officers. He was characterized by a later Assistant Surgeon General as "solid, dependable, and industrious," qualities "more needed at that time in the history of the organization than great brilliance or originality."[26] While he did not achieve bacteriological discoveries himself, Kinyoun was obviously captured by the vision of research as a potent weapon against disease. In 1894 he again went to Europe, this time to study Emile Roux's method of producing diphtheria vaccine. Impressed with the potential transferability of the process, Kinyoun wrote:

> The results obtained by Professor E. M. Roux of the Pasteur Institute in the treatment of cases of diphtheria are so astounding that at first one is almost compelled to ask oneself, "Is this possible?" But when the methods are known and the array of statistics are given, there can hardly remain a trace of doubt. . . . It appears that at last we have found a method which is not only good in one disease, but the principles of the method can be applied to many. It has opened up a new field for work in infectious diseases.[27]

Kinyoun was also aware, however, that the production and sale of the sera being developed offered economic profits that would attract charlatans as well as producers with integrity. "There are many questions regarding the toxins, and the production of antitoxin, still unsolved," he noted in 1895, "and it will require time to define them."[28] He went on to observe: "Many persons will, during the ensuing year, commence to prepare the serum as a business enterprise, and there will, without doubt, be worthless articles called antitoxin thrown upon the market. All serum intended for sale should be made or tested by competent persons."[29] Kinyoun's call for regulation of these "biologics," as they came to be known, was finally heeded by Congress in 1902 after a number of deaths from contaminated antitoxin.[30] The development of standard strength biologicals and the testing of products manufactured for sale became one of the major congressionally designated obligations of the Laboratory in the first three decades of the twentieth century.

In 1891 the Hygienic Laboratory was moved to Washington, D.C., and given quarters in the Butler Building near the Capitol.[31] Very little original research was performed by the staff of the Laboratory in these early years of its existence. Its instruments and Kinyoun's expertise were utilized in a variety of ways, however. After his trip to Europe in 1894, for example, Kinyoun prepared diphtheria antitoxin in Washington and taught state and local health officials the new techniques. His first students were representatives of the state boards of North Carolina, Minnesota, and Maine, and of the local boards of Norfolk, Virginia; Cumberland, Maryland; and Montgomery County, Maryland.[32]

Kinyoun was also called upon to aid health officials of the District of Columbia and to provide advice to Congress. In 1894 the District board of health requested bacteriological analysis of water wells. Kinyoun's analysis demonstrated that about 90 percent were contaminated with sewage.[33] Two years later an epidemic of typhoid fever struck Washington. Local health authorities investigated, but the Laboratory performed all the bacteriological work.[34] The United States Congress in 1894 called upon the Laboratory to examine the ventilation of the House of Representatives. Kinyoun found that the air of that chamber contained illuminating gas from leaking gas pipes. The air was "further vitiated by persons smoking," and the carpet on the floor of the House and in the galleries had in some places been "saturated with tobacco expectoration," which tended "to make it odorous."[35] Similar ventilation studies were made for Congress throughout the early twentieth century.

The Laboratory's status as a useful but clearly secondary tool to the larger public health mission may also be seen in the fact that Kinyoun was assigned regular Service duties during his tenure as Laboratory director. He supervised quarantine restrictions during the 1892 cholera epidemic. He prepared exhibits for the World's Columbian Exposition in 1893. Such duties restricted his laboratory work, but his devotion to the Laboratory that he had established set precedents for his successors. Determined to educate Service officers in laboratory techniques, Kinyoun began a "systematic course of instruction in bacteriology" during the winter of 1894.[36] The school was continued and expanded by his successors. Milton J. Rosenau, director of the Laboratory from 1899 until 1909, used the course as a screening process by which to identify potential career researchers.[37] In 1914 it was broadened to include instruction in zoology, pharmacy, and chemistry, and in 1915 original research projects were assigned as part of the curriculum.[38] After World War I, nonlaboratory public health procedures were introduced into the course.[39]

By 1899 Kinyoun had fallen from favor with Supervising Surgeon Walter Wyman. It is unclear exactly why Wyman decided to replace Kinyoun, but the founder of the Laboratory was transferred to San Francisco and became embroiled in the political debacle of the 1901 plague outbreak in that city. Shortly thereafter he resigned from the Service, feeling "he had not been given the backing he deserved" in San Francisco.[40] He became director of H. K. Mulford Laboratories and later accepted the chair of pathology at George Washington University.[41] The man chosen to succeed Kinyoun was Milton J. Rosenau.[42] Having taken his M.D. at the University of Pennsylvania in 1889 when he was only twenty years old, Rosenau joined the Service and was quickly recognized by Walter Wyman as a bright young officer with research potential. Rosenau was assigned to be Kinyoun's assistant in the Laboratory from time to time and was just thirty years old when he became its new director.

As Rosenau began his directorship, the United States was recovering from the Spanish American War, an episode that first tested the usefulness of the Hygienic Laboratory in a national crisis. The Laboratory's services were put at military disposal and were used primarily for bacteriological diagnosis of infectious diseases, especially typhoid fever, in an effort to prevent their entrance into the United States.[43] The success with which the job was done demonstrated the value of a government laboratory that could be immediately utilized in an emergency. Over thirty thousand troops were inspected for disease as they reentered the United States. Many were sick, but no wholesale importation of diseases occurred to endanger the population. Supervising Surgeon Wyman commented in his annual report for 1898 on the Service's role in this conflict:

> In closing this report, which is made at the close of a season notable by reason of the great apprehension which was felt at its beginning lest epidemic disaster should fall upon the country as a result of military and naval operations against Cuba, and notable, too, in the fact that no such results followed, I deem it proper to invite attention to the grave responsibilities and unusual exertions, continued throughout the summer and fall, which were imposed upon the Marine Hospital Service.[44]

Wyman, who was a master at sensing the politically opportune time to press for an expansion of the Service's role, took advantage of the appreciation felt toward Service officers and the Laboratory to gain further recognition for both. Two factors prodded him to action. Throughout the 1890s delegations of physicians and public health leaders had continued to press the case for a separate national department of health. In 1895, for example, a delegation from the New York Academy of Medicine came to Washington to testify for a bill based on the plan Henry I. Bowditch had presented to the American Medical Association in 1875.[45] None of these bills had gotten out of committee, but they were potential threats to the Service's hegemony in federal public health activities. Furthermore, the yellow fever investigations after the Spanish American War stirred up controversy between the medical corps of the War Department and some members of the Marine Hospital Service. The latter rejected the mosquito vector theory of yellow fever proposed by the War Department, believing *Bacillus icteroides* to be the probable cause.[46] The mosquito vector concept, Wyman wrote in his 1901 annual report, was "scientifically, an entirely new subject, and the relation of insects to the conveyance of diseases needs more definite proof than simple observation or sup-position."[47] This incident, which proved embarrassing to the Service after the mosquito vector theory was demonstrated to be correct, was at the turn of the century awkward only because Congress was not pleased to see "two great departments of the Government . . . at each other's throat upon a scientific subject."[48] With pressure for a separate department of health from outside groups and controversy between existing agencies, it is not surprising that Wyman chose to press the case for expansion of the Service while Congress was fa-vorably inclined toward it.

In 1901 Wyman guided legislation through Congress that, for the first time in law, recognized the Hygienic Laboratory by providing it with thirty-five thousand dollars for a separate building and authorizing it to investigate "infectious and contagious diseases, and matters per-taining to the public health."[49] This organic act was buried in a sundry civil appropriations bill, but most of the scientific bureaus of the gov-ernment in the late nineteenth century had been created in the same manner.[50] The 1901 act, like many others affecting the Service, served primarily to legitimate what was already accomplished in fact. The investigation of infectious diseases had been occurring for some years. The appropriation for a separate building was welcomed as a means to expand out of the cramped Butler Building quarters. The new building, occupied in 1904, was located at Twenty-fifth and E Streets, Northwest, in Washington, D.C.

In 1902 Wyman won another major battle in his drive to make the Service the legitimate public health bureau of the federal government. He took advantage of the concern generated by the disagreement over the cause of yellow fever to get a reorganization bill before Congress. According to G. Lloyd Magruder, a Washington physician, the idea for a reorganization bill began in Magruder's office during a conference with Wisconsin senator John C. Spooner, a member of the Senate Committee on Public Health and National Quarantine.[51] Searching for a solution to the problem of conflicting reports on scientific subjects by government bureaus, Magruder said he suggested to Spooner: "Let us have a clearing house; the hygienic laboratory should be the clearing house. We have some of the greatest scientists in the country connected with the Government today and if you make a clearing house of that hygienic laboratory, composed of the best scientists of the Government, with some men from outside, you will get something that can not be attacked."[52] Spooner agreed, according to Magruder's account of the meeting, and asked Wyman to initiate legislation to accomplish this.

In 1902 the bill that Wyman drew up was enacted. It did more than enlarge the Hygienic Laboratory; it provided for a complete reorganization of the Service.[53] The act authorized the renaming of the Marine Hospital Service, adding the prefix "Public Health." This change enhanced the Service's claim to being a legitimate federal department of health. Under this new Public Health and Marine Hospital Service, Wyman was designated Surgeon General rather than Supervising Surgeon. The new title gave the office a status more in line with that of the leaders of the military medical services, although the congressional committee responsible for the bill stated that the change was made merely because the designation "Supervising" was cumbersome.[54] This sensitivity of Congress to any implication that the Service might receive military status, moreover, resulted in the committee's elimination of one section of the bill providing military ranks for Service officers in time of war.[55] The measure also provided for an annual meeting of state and territorial health officers with the Surgeon General, one goal of the 1875 Bowditch plan. This provision, which was considered "by all means the most important section in the bill," was a step toward bridging the longstanding states rights chasm that had hampered cooperation between state and federal health authorities.[56]

With regard to the original desire for better coordination of government scientific research activities, the new law made several revisions in the organization of the Service. It authorized a Division of Scientific Research to coordinate all the research activities within the Service. In 1902 these included the work of the Hygienic Laboratory and of the Plague Laboratory in San Francisco, cooperative work on yellow fever with researchers in universities, and cooperative work with Montana State health authorities on Rocky Mountain spotted fever. In order to promote research in infectious diseases, the law also authorized the Service to collect information on the incidence of morbidity, mortality, and other vital statistics. Unfortunately, the act did not include an appropriation to fund this provision, so this authority of the Service, which overlapped the vital statistics work of the Bureau of the Census, was not exercised.

The 1902 law also addressed the Hygienic Laboratory directly. One provision, another item in the old Bowditch plan, established an eight-member Advisory Board for the Laboratory. This board included three "competent experts" detailed from the Army, Navy, and the Bureau of Animal Industry. In addition, five other members "skilled in laboratory work in its relation to the public health, and not in the regular employ of the Government" were designated to be appointed by the Surgeon General. The mission of the board was to bring "the national laboratory into scientific touch with most of the large private or corporate laboratories in the United States" and permit "the coordination of scientific work and opportunity to avoid unnecessary duplication of scientific investigation."[57] Board members, who included the distinguished William H. Welch of the Johns Hopkins University Medical School as first chairman, offered advice to the Surgeon General that was perceived as extremely helpful in the work of the Laboratory. In 1908 and 1909, for example, the board encouraged the Hygienic Laboratory to continue and broaden a study it had begun on typhoid fever in the District of Columbia because, as they noted, it was "really national in character."[58] This investigation was later described as "one of the most valuable contributions which America has made to epidemiology."[59] Information gathered in the District proved applicable to later campaigns against typhoid in both rural and urban areas.[60]

A final provision of the 1902 act authorized the creation of three new divisions within the Laboratory. The existing staff was designated the Division of Pathology and Bacteriology, a name that reflected the major concerns and areas of achievement of nineteenth-century medicine. The new Divisions of Chemistry, Pharmacology, and Zoology were sorely needed, but the Commissioned Officers Corps of the Service lacked personnel trained in those areas who could direct the research. Because of this, the law allowed the Service to hire "competent persons" to take charge of the new divisions; these men soon became known as "Professors." It was stipulated that the head of the Division of Pathology and Bacteriology and the director of the Laboratory—in practice the same person—be commissioned officers. An early draft of the bill that became the 1902 law had called for commissioning the Professors also. Because of "objection to this by the officers" of the Service, however, the law ultimately stated that they would be Civil Service employees.[61]

The Commissioned Officers Corps had been created in 1889 with the goal of establishing a professional body of officers for the Service.[62] These men were available on short notice for detail at any location where they were needed. The examinations for admission to the corps were rigorous, and promotions were earned only after years of service. All members of the corps were physicians, and no distinction was made between clinicians and nonclinical research physicians. The opposition of the corps to the admission of nonmedical personnel was probably based both on professional pride and on a desire to keep the corps as it was, a mobile body. Appointments that were permanent in one location, as those of division directors in the Hygienic Laboratory were likely to be, might well cause dissension among officers ordered to undesirable duty stations. The discrepancies in pay and perquisites between Professors and commissioned officers caused by this provision, however, led to a high turnover among the distinguished scientists hired to direct some of the new divisions.

From both a political and a scientific standpoint the laws of 1901 and 1902 marked a watershed in the history of the Hygienic Laboratory. Politically they legitimated the research function of the Laboratory and provided a mechanism for orderly expansion. Scientifically they allowed the Laboratory to enter the mainstream of biomedical research. The new director, Milton Rosenau, presided over the implementation of the new law. In order to provoke more concern with research, he inaugurated in 1902 weekly meetings of the staff "to stimulate interest in the literature."[63] Each researcher was assigned certain journals from which to present critical reviews on timely research developments. These gatherings became known in 1906 as the "Journal Club." In later years each division established its own journal club as the volume and specialization of the literature mounted.[64] Saturday morning inspections of all laboratory stations became mandatory in 1903. Laboratory personnel, who worked a forty-eight-hour week, handled numerous highly contagious organisms, and these inspections kept to a minimum the likelihood of contracting the diseases being studied.[65]

In 1900 Rosenau began publication of the *Bulletin of the Hygienic Laboratory*, which contained articles of a more arcane scientific nature than the Service's *Public Health Reports*. The *Bulletins* were yet another example of expansion within the Laboratory before approval by statute; it was not until 1905 that Congress belatedly made formal provision for publication of these documents. By the mid-1920s over 140 *Bulletins* had been published.[66]

In 1909 Rosenau resigned from the Laboratory to become chairman of the Department of Preventive Medicine and Hygiene at Harvard University. He was succeeded by John F. Anderson, who served as director from 1909 until 1915 and then by George W. McCoy, who served as director from 1915 until 1938.[67] Anderson and McCoy built on the organizational pattern established by Rosenau. The Laboratory remained a small facility, and the director knew each researcher and his or her work individually.

The research program of the Hygienic Laboratory launched under the 1901 and 1902 acts reflected the major lines of research in the early twentieth century. Most of these were elaborations of work begun in the nineteenth century. One of the oldest types of scientific research, for example, was the collection and classification of flora and fauna. Within the Hygienic Laboratory this type of work was continued by the Division of Zoology and its first director, Charles Wardell Stiles. The first division director to be named for the three new divisions created by the 1902 act, Stiles began a tenure of twenty-nine years on August 16, 1902.[68] Stiles came to the post from the Bureau of Animal Industry, where in May 1902 he had described a new species of hookworm that came to bear his name, *Necator americanus* (Stiles). He had received reports that the worm was found in Georgia and correctly deduced that it, rather then malaria, was the cause of much anemia found in the South.

Stiles "was not a speculative thinker; his strength lay rather in observation."[69] Zoology in the early twentieth century had need of people with such talent because there was still much identification and classification work to be done. During his tenure in the Hygienic Laboratory, Stiles prepared with staff member Albert Hassall an *Index-Catalog of Medical and Veterinary Zoology.* The *Index-Catalog,* supplemented by a series of *Key Catalogs* on insects, parasites, protozoa, crustacea, and arachnids, has been termed by James H. Cassedy "a scientific and bibliographic accomplishment comparable in magnitude and importance to the *Index-Catalogue* of the Surgeon General's library prepared by John Shaw Billings."[70] Stiles also served on the International Commission of Zoological Nomenclature, which negotiated the internationally recognized scientific names for various species. While accomplishing this bibliographic and administrative work, he served as scientific advisor to the Rockefeller Hookworm Commission, a capacity in which he is better known. He traveled extensively, gathering statistical data, educating health professionals about hookworm disease, lecturing to the public, and designing privies.

The work of the Division of Zoology was in the nineteenth century tradition of natural history: observation, description, classification. Furthermore, it was exceedingly useful and practical. This was the kind of research that the public could understand and Congress could easily justify supporting. Information gleaned about hookworms or insects could be used directly in public action to improve health. The major trends in medical research in the late nineteenth century, however, were moving beyond empirical work. New methods and procedures directed the course of research toward analysis, synthesis, and the posing of some theoretical models. On an organizational plane, this meant the rise of team research and the correlation of different fields. In the laboratory it meant increased reliance on quantitative methods, the use of experimental animals, and the development of new instruments that permitted the acquisition of more accurate data.

The field of bacteriology was the first to enjoy success with this new approach. Louis Pasteur and Robert Koch conducted pioneer studies that spurred researchers to look for bacterial causes for almost all diseases. Using the microscope, staining methods, improved culture media, and experimental animals, bacteriologists discovered the microbial agents responsible for diphtheria, cholera, tuberculosis, and a number of other scourges. Vaccines were produced in animals to combat some of these diseases, while other maladies proved more intractable. Identification of certain organisms in water and milk supplies, the discovery of insect vectors for disease, and the recognition of human carriers who harbored a germ but did not become ill—all these lines of research provided information that could be used to combat or contain infectious diseases.[71]

Because of their dramatic threat to public health, infectious diseases were the first to be studied in the Hygienic Laboratory. In the first four decades of the twentieth century, the Division of Pathology and Bacteriology made major contributions to the study of over thirty infectious diseases.[72] The Laboratory's study of typhoid fever in the Progressive Era has already been mentioned. Two other notable contributions will point out the kind of work pursued. While conducting work on plague between 1908 and 1911, George McCoy, who, as stated, would become director of the Laboratory in 1915, identified a species of bacteria (*Bacterium tularense*) in ground squirrels that he named after the county in which he was working, Tulare, California. In 1919 Edward Francis began further work on this bacterium and subsequently identified a wholly new disease, tularemia. This was an early instance "in which American investigators had identified a new infectious disease of man, isolated its causative agent, and determined the sources of infection and methods of transmission to man."[73] The work of bacteriologist Alice C. Evans on undulant fever was also of special note. Evans, who with Ida A. Bengtson was one of the first women employed on the scientific staff of the Laboratory, determined that the organisms that caused abortive fever in cattle and Malta fever in man were variations of the same bacterium. Her work resulted in the identification of undulant fever as a human form of abortive fever, and she traced its transmission to contaminated milk.[74] This hastened the spread of the pasteurization movement in the United States.

Bacteriologists, including those in the Hygienic Laboratory, concentrated primarily on the action of the so-called microbes on plants and larger animals, including humans. Other researchers at this time were developing methods to examine the chemistry of biological systems. The tools of the new discipline—biochemistry—that emerged proved to be the keys to some of the most important advances in medical science in the twentieth century.[75] Biochemists, for example, developed specific adsorbants to separate closely related substances without chemical change. The new adsorbants, primarily synthetic resins as opposed to the old standard adsorbant charcoal, assisted the identification of substances by chromotography, a process of filtering materials so that their component parts separate in layers as they pass through the filters. Theodor Svedberg, a professor in Upsala, Sweden, utilized centrifugal machines employed in the sugar and starch industries since the mid-nineteenth century to develop the "ultracentrifuge" that made possible the identification of large, heavy molecules. Arne Tiselius, another researcher in Svedberg's laboratory, exploited the property of molecules to migrate under the influence of an electrical potential to develop "electrophoresis" as a method to determine the size and shape of molecules. Biochemists also pointed out the necessity for careful control of temperature and factors such as hydrogen ion concentration in experimental work.

Such biochemical methods—and these represent just a sample of notable developments—were embraced by physiologists and bacteriologists.[76] Early in the century the three basic blood groups were identified: A, B, and O. An understanding of blood as a colloidal substance and advances in colloidal chemistry further elucidated the characteristics of this vital body fluid. Biochemical work on respiration, which was understood as a form of combustion, was also conducted before 1925. Moreover, biochemical methods made possible the work most easily defined as twentieth century in origin, research into vitamins.[77] The concept of essential food factors was accepted early in the century—the word *vitamine* was coined in 1911. Shortly thereafter, researchers in America and Europe identified an alphabet of substances that in small quantities prevented scurvy, pellagra, and rickets, to cite but three examples. Other lines of research in biochemistry and physiology focused on the action of hormones and enzymes in the body. Japanese researchers uncovered the natural healing enzymes in plants and extended speculation about their presence in animals as well. By 1940 work in vitamins, hormones, and enzymes was converging. The description of many metabolic pathways had been accomplished, and identification of hormones as body regulators and enzymes as catalysts had been established. This work allowed investigators after World War II to begin to unravel the mystery of the molecular activities within the cell.

The first chief of the Division of Chemistry in the Hygienic Laboratory, Joseph Hoeing Kastle, was representative of the chemists adopting the new methods of biochemistry.[78] His research on oxidases was notable; he also worked on a chemical method to identify and estimate the amount of hydrochloric acid in the stomach.[79] The reagent he identified for this method came to be known as "Kastle's reagent." In 1907 Kastle turned his attention to the chemistry of the blood. His division worked on the development of a "hemoglobinometer" for measuring the amount of hemoglobin in the blood, "which it is believed," he wrote, "will be a distinct advance over any instrument of the kind now in use."[80] Indeed, the instrument became the standard device for measuring hemoglobin for several decades.

At the same time that biochemical methods were yielding fruitful information in some fields, an enlightened empiricism was providing additional knowledge without benefit of theoretical understanding. Statistical analysis became a powerful tool for use in clinical trials of new therapeutic agents and in epidemiological studies, both of which were conducted on an empirical basis.[81] Results obtained in this manner successfully informed many treatment and control programs. The Hygienic Laboratory investigation of typhoid fever in the District of Columbia was one notable example. Pharmaceutical research, likewise, proceeded with some success in an empirical fashion. Especially after the discovery of the sulfa drugs in the 1930s, such practical work actually stimulated the creation of theory.[82] Indeed, perhaps more than in any other field, the complexities of drug research required the combined use of biochemical methodology and creative empiricism. Raymond F. Bacon, director of the Mellon Institute for Industrial Research, described the state of the pharmaceutical art in 1914:

> The teachings of physical chemistry have led to the study of the conditions of absorption of drugs by the various cells and tissue juices of the body, of the part played therein by osmosis, by electrolytic dissociation, by mass, and especially by the colloidal character of substances concerned in metabolism. Such study associated with biological chemistry has pointed the way for a fuller understanding of the complexities of the processes that are comprised in the physiological action of drugs.[83]

In the Hygienic Laboratory, the background of Reid Hunt, the first chief of the Division of Pharmacology, enabled the Laboratory to become a leader in scientific pharmacology.[84] Hunt had studied physiology with William H. Howell at the Johns Hopkins University and spent a summer in Chicago with Jacques Loeb and Julius Stieglitz applying chemical methods to biological problems. His first major position was on the faculty of pharmacology at Johns Hopkins, where he worked with John J. Abel, the foremost pharmacologist of the time. In 1903 and 1904, while his laboratory at the Hygienic Laboratory was being prepared, Hunt worked at the Institut für experimentelle Therapie at Frankfurt am Main, under Paul Ehrlich, who exercised a strong influence on his scientific interests.

Hunt's major interest was the powerful biological action of acetylcholine on blood pressure. In 1906 he published with R. de M. Taveau a biological method for the assay of choline.[85] He was also interested in the effects of alcohol and in 1902 alerted the American medical profession to the toxicity of methyl alcohol. His "brilliant descriptions" of the pharmacology and toxicity of methyl and ethyl alcohols became of great importance later during the Prohibition period.[86] Moreover, Hunt had discovered while working with Paul Ehrlich that mice fed thyroid tolerated an amount of acetonitrile several times the lethal dose. Known officially as the "acetonitrile test for thyroid activity," the practical test he developed from this observation became commonly known as the "Reid Hunt reaction."[87]

These examples of research conducted under the auspices of the 1901 and 1902 acts demonstrate the vigor with which the Laboratory's staff pursued their interests within the pragmatic bounds required of a federal agency. Under these laws, physicians and scientists in the Laboratory were able to inaugurate investigations that placed them at the cutting edge of medical research. Many who began their careers during this period later reaped a wide variety of honors. By 1940 twelve members of the Laboratory had received the distinction of being starred in various editions of *American Men of Science*. Starred scientists represented the one thousand men in each edition whose contributions were deemed to be most important. Five members of the Laboratory also received the Sedgwick Memorial Medal, the highest honor in the public health field, awarded by the American Public Health Association.[88] The popular scientific writer Paul de Kruif also featured the staff of the Twenty-fifth and E Streets, Northwest, laboratory—what he called "the little red brick building on the hill"— in several of his books.[89]

In addition to praise from the American scientific community, the Hygienic Laboratory received international recognition in the early twentieth century. One Washington physician, for example, recounted this experience at the Pasteur Institute in Paris, where he had gone in 1909 to obtain information on milk control in Paris:

> I was in the institution itself, and they said: "Doctor, you are fortunate in arriving here at this time; the secretary of the International Institute of Hygiene is in the room and he can give you the information you want. We have no information in regard to the bacteriological flora of milk." I went to the International Institute with the secretary. He took down from the shelves this book, Bulletin 56 [of the Hygienic Laboratory]. He said: "This is the greatest book in the world on the subject; we look to it all the time."[90]

Such a standing prompted Surgeon General Walter Wyman to write glowingly in his 1911 annual report: "The Hygienic Laboratory is acknowledged by all to be now one of the five or six greatest research laboratories in the world. The amount and class of work turned out of the laboratory is second to none."[91]

Enthusiasm for the work of the Hygienic Laboratory must be understood within the limits imposed upon it by congressional mandate. The budget of the Laboratory in this period was small; indeed, it was not until 1907 that its research allocation, fifteen thousand dollars, was mentioned separately in the annual report of the Surgeon General. In that same year the staff of the Laboratory numbered thirty-two, which included technicians, clerks, and laboratory aides.[92] Researchers were restricted by law to investigate "infectious and contagious diseases" and were not free to pursue their personal research interests as were their counterparts in universities. John W. Kerr, who served as the director of the Division of Scientific Research in the Service from 1905 until 1918, noted in a memoir Congress's demanding oversight of virtually every penny expended and commented that because of this the public servant could not expect to initiate expensive, open-ended research programs.[93] Such restrictions were not challenged by members of the Laboratory staff, but as the first decade of the twentieth century progressed, the results of their research led some of them into areas not expressly covered by the Laboratory's enabling legislation. By 1912 Congress would find it necessary again to address the proper scope of this emerging federal biomedical research facility.

TWO
Institutionalization and Development in the Progressive Era

As the scientific work of the service proceeds, its importance
becomes more and more apparent. It is safe to say that the
results obtained from one line of study alone have been of many times
greater value than the entire appropriation for studies of public health
matters for the year.
John Kerr, 1915

I n his 1907 annual report, Surgeon General Walter Wyman remarked that the scientific work of the Hygienic Laboratory had
"excited widespread and favorable comment among scientists
and public health officials both in this country and abroad."[1] He
was writing during the period of rapid expansion of the Laboratory in
the Progressive Era. It was during these years that the Laboratory
secured for itself a permanent foothold in the federal government
through its research work and regulatory activities. It was also in this
period that the Laboratory began to feel constrained by the limits
imposed by its enabling legislation.

Progressive Era regulatory legislation significantly aided the insti-
tutionalization of federal scientific bureaus that had been created in
the nineteenth century. The public, outraged by the exposés in muckraking publications, perceived the regulatory laws to be beneficial and
accepted the employment of additional scientific specialists by the
government as a necessary part of enforcement. The 1906 Meat
Inspection Act and Pure Food and Drugs Act, for example, had been
hastened to passage by the publication of Upton Sinclair's novel *The
Jungle* and Samuel Hopkins Adams's series in *Collier's* on patent medicines, "The Great American Fraud."[2] An enlarged cadre of federal
scientists to assist in the enforcement of these laws seemed a small
price to pay for the benefits received, even to a public traditionally
suspicious of any entrenched federal bureaucracy.

The Hygienic Laboratory became a regulatory agency four years
before the Pure Food and Drugs Act was passed and with less fanfare
than that better known legislation received. In 1902 the Laboratory
was charged with the enforcement of the earliest piece of Progressive

Era health legislation, the Biologics Control Act. "Biologics" or "biologicals" at that time referred to vaccines and antitoxins that were injected into the human body to prevent or treat disease. They were produced by injecting an animal, usually a horse, with pathogens of some disease and later extracting serum from the animal that contained antibodies to the disease. The potential benefits were great from smallpox vaccine and diphtheria antitoxin, two of the earliest biological products produced, but the hazards involved in production were equally great. Horses had to be kept free from disease; stables and horses alike had to be kept scrupulously clean; knowledgable bacteriologists had to supervise the preparation of the serum under sterile conditions. Improper technique at any point in the process could endanger the life of the patient treated with the product. The need for a law to regulate the production of vaccines and sera had been recognized by the Laboratory's first director, Joseph J. Kinyoun, as early as 1895. And although many other people had also been concerned about unregulated production of biologicals, by 1900 little had been done. It required the widespread reporting of disasters from contaminated biologicals, especially a tragedy in which thirteen children in St. Louis died from contaminated diphtheria antitoxin, to prod Congress into action in 1902.[3]

Under the Biologics Control Act, which became effective August 21, 1903, the Laboratory's Division of Pathology and Bacteriology annually inspected the laboratories of manufacturers of the products, testing the preparations for purity and, as standard strengths were developed, for potency as well. The division issued licenses to firms that met these standards. It first produced a standard diphtheria antitoxin, which was introduced April 1, 1905. Two years later a standard unit of tetanus antitoxin was defined, based on a standard potency of tetanus toxin. Development of these and subsequent standards "saved the pharmaceutical industry much research and development money."[4] Enforcement of the standards was conducted with tact and firmness, and relations were cordial between corporate manufacturers of the sera and the Hygienic Laboratory. In 1908 the examination of sera was extended to those prepared by state and local boards of health when requested by those authorities. In the first year six states and one territory requested tests.[5] Officials from state and local boards continued to visit the Hygienic Laboratory to be instructed in bacteriology and to examine the laboratory facilities. Representatives of serum laboratories and public health officials from foreign countries also came to the Laboratory, including researchers from China, Australia, Czechoslovakia, Norway, and Poland.[6] The techniques of sera preparation, particularly those to produce "vaccine virus" for smallpox vaccinations, always excited "a great deal of interest and favorable comment from visitors."[7]

By 1908, twenty-four establishments were licensed to produce biologics. These firms included large pharmaceutical houses like Parke, Davis, and Company; small state health departments; private institutes such as the John McCormick Memorial Institute in Chicago; and foreign manufacturers such as the Pasteur Institute in France and Burroughs, Wellcome, and Company in England.[8] The fact that leading foreign pharmaceutical houses adopted the standard units prepared by the Hygienic Laboratory attested to the high regard in which the work of the Laboratory was held.

Problems encountered with vaccine regulation stimulated original research in the division. In 1906 Milton Rosenau and John F. Anderson published the first of their pioneering studies on anaphylaxis, "A Study of the Cause of Sudden Death Following the Injection of Horse Serum."[9] Anderson continued the work after Rosenau resigned from the Service. Expanding his study to general cases of hypersensitivity, Anderson and his colleague W. H. Frost published an article in 1910 in which the word *allergin* appeared in medical literature for the first time.[10]

Through its work with biologicals, the Laboratory also became involved with evaluating new products. Members of the Laboratory staff had studied the Pasteur treatment for rabies in the late nineteenth century but dropped further studies of the disease because the Pasteur treatment was effective. In the early twentieth century, however, this treatment could be obtained in the United States only at so-called Pasteur Institutes, a few widely scattered clinics that prepared the injections. In 1908 some scientists claimed to have developed new serum and virus treatments for rabies that were different from the classical Pasteur treatment. The Laboratory resumed its study of rabies at this time in order to evaluate the new products' claims. The Division of Pathology and Bacteriology discounted the new products, but in the course of its own work developed "a method of preserving glycerinated spinal cords of rabbits," allowing them to be more easily shipped to state health officials having laboratory facilities.[11] This greatly increased the distribution of the treatment because "exposed persons in any part of the country had to travel no further than to their own State health office."[12] The Laboratory also began offering the Pasteur treatment to any person in the District of Columbia bitten by a rabid animal. Begun April 28, 1908, these treatments were continued until January 21, 1921, when there were enough local treatment centers available to make the Laboratory's involvement unnecessary.[13]

The expansion of research in the Hygienic Laboratory that accompanied its regulatory function as well as that conducted under the auspices of the 1901 and 1902 laws sometimes led staff members into areas not specifically addressed by the mandate to investigate "infectious and contagious diseases." For example, consistent findings that water pollution was the source of outbreaks of typhoid fever had led to demands for further investigation of the pollution of interstate waterways. The American Medical Association called for the Public Health and Marine Hospital Service to "formulate and enforce necessary regulations to prevent pollution of the waterways."[14] Members of the Laboratory staff were interested in the problem, but it was unclear whether the general subject of water pollution was included in the congressionally mandated mission of the Laboratory. Two other lines of research that also raised questions were Charles W. Stiles's work on hookworm, which has already been mentioned, and the investigations of Joseph Goldberger and others on pellagra. The pellagra investigations, requested by southern state health authorities, had begun initially on the assumption that a bacterium was the probable cause of the disease. Goldberger's controlled studies, particularly in South Carolina, Georgia, and Mississippi, convinced him that it was of a dietary origin instead.[15]

Research into water pollution, hookworm, and pellagra, of course, had broad social implications. Commercial interests were affronted by the water pollution studies; the investigations of hookworm and pellagra pointed up the results of poverty in the South. Consequently, Service officials and some congressmen occasionally differed over whether the Service was exceeding its authority by pursuing research in these areas. Assistant Surgeon General John Kerr, who was also director of the Division of Scientific Research, believed that the Service was within its mandate. He interpreted broadly the 1901 act providing for research into "infectious and contagious diseases and matters pertaining to the public health."[16] Illinois congressman James R. Mann, a physician and consistent supporter of the Service, disagreed. He believed that clarifying legislation was needed because there existed "a question as to whether they [the Public Health and Marine Hospital Service] really have jurisdiction to make investigations of such diseases as pellagra, hookworm, and some new diseases which have come up."[17]

While this question was being debated, a second problem area arose concerning the pay and perquisites of Service employees. The remuneration of commissioned officers and of Hygienic Laboratory Professors, the nonmedical scientists who headed the Divisions of Zoology, Chemistry, and Pharmacology, was a longstanding concern. In 1889, when the Commissioned Officers Corps was established, the pay of commissioned officers had been made the same as that of Army and Navy medical officers. Over the years, however, increases in pay had been granted to military physicians but not to those in the Public Health and Marine Hospital Service. In addition, military officers were promoted more rapidly, and this in effect also increased their pay further. Other perquisites available to Army and Navy officers, such as purchasing goods at post exchanges, were not available to the officers of the Service. The result was that military physicians received from $200 to $2,000 per year more than their Service counterparts.[18] This situation caused the Service difficulties in recruiting new officers and retaining existing ones.

The discrepancies in pay and perquisites between Service officers and Hygienic Laboratory Professors have been mentioned previously. Although commissioned officers had objected to the commissioning of nonmedical scientists, the Senate committee contemplating the 1902 act had "deemed it important" that "during the upbuilding of the work, there should be freedom to attract by adequate compensation those best qualified."[19] Therefore, when the Service was negotiating with Charles Wardell Stiles, first of the Professors hired, "it was arranged to obtain the salaries of ten leading universities for positions in this and similar lines and average those salaries as the 'base pay.' "[20] Moreover, as an inducement to join the Laboratory, Wyman had promised the Professors that they would be "entitled to all the privileges of the Service which the commissioned officers enjoyed, including accumulative leave, and waiting orders," the Service's terminology for disability retirement.[21]

Wyman, unfortunately, had overstepped his authority in making such offers. Under the Civil Service regulations governing the Professors, annual leave could not be accumulated, and scant protection was offered for a work-related disability. The Professors complained bitterly about the misrepresentation of their status, and Surgeon General Wyman agreed to seek changes in the law to elevate them to a level equal to professorships at West Point. By 1909, however, nothing had changed. In a letter to the Surgeon General in February 1909, Stiles and his colleagues Reid Hunt and Joseph Kastle outlined their complaints and pointed out that each had "declined positions elsewhere" on the basis of promised improvements.[22]

Both of these research and in-house personnel concerns, however, became enmeshed in a third problem, the larger question of federal public health policy. Leading figures in American public health were dismayed by the fact that many European nations had established departments or ministries of health in the late nineteenth century while

the United States had no such central body. Reform of medical education and medical licensure was proceeding in the first decade of the
twentieth century, but at the same time, irregular medical sects and
patent medicine interests continued to flourish. To those who es-
poused scientific medicine, this situation was anathema.

The approaches taken to this problem by leading public health figures
had not changed significantly since the National Board of Health fiasco
in the 1880s. Leaders of the Public Health and Marine Hospital Service
hoped to expand their own agency into a more powerful public health
department, but other public health leaders yearned for a separate
agency. These points of view clashed head-on in the Progressive Era
when a new campaign was launched for a national department of health.
The research and personnel concerns of the Hygienic Laboratory
quickly became subordinate issues, because from 1906 to 1912 the
Service was again forced to defend its primacy in the federal health
establishment. On this occasion the opposition was formidable; Wyndham Miles observed that this Progressive Era movement marshalled
support from more prominent Americans than any other attempt since
that time.[23]

The rhetoric and strategy of the Progressive Era campaign owed
much to the conservation movement around the turn of the century.[24]
Inspired by the enthusiastic leadership of President Theodore Roosevelt, conservationists advocated the planned use and scientific management of all the nation's resources. Health, to them, was a precious
national resource not to be overlooked. The movement to conserve
human resources was led by two economists, J. Pease Norton and
Irving Fisher, both of Yale University. Because of their professional
interests, much of the rhetoric of the campaign was couched in terms
of business management, so statistics abounded on the "cost effec-
tiveness" of preventing disease and the overall contribution this would
make to "national efficiency." In this approach they were no different
from other Progressive Era reformers who believed that a major goal
of their work was to produce an efficient, rational society.[25]

In 1906, the same year crusaders succeeded in obtaining legislation
regulating food and drug purity, Norton spoke before the American
Association for the Advancement of Science (AAAS) about the high
economic cost of illness and premature death. He recommended the
establishment of a department of health that would "take all measures
calculated, in the judgment of experts, to decrease deaths, to decrease
sickness, and to increase physical and mental efficiency of citizens."
The proposed department would include a bureau of research pos-
sessing laboratories whose "vital problem" would be "to make new

discoveries of value at a rapid rate." Norton continued, describing how this goal would be accomplished:

> New discoveries or inventions in general depend on the number of exceptional men in a society capable of such work. . . . The necessity of employing experts cannot be overemphasized. . . . The organization in vogue among modern business corporations and the practice of playing off against each other several experts engaged in independently solving the same problem should be adopted. That which can be accomplished through organization of the world's exceptional men under the lash of failures and stimulus of great rewards is of vast magnitude. [26]

Norton's talk, with its optimism about what could be accomplished by well-managed experts, stimulated the AAAS to appoint a "Committee of One Hundred on National Health" to study the subject and promote enabling legislation. [27]

The committee, whose members included such prominent Americans as Jane Addams and Luther Burbank, took its task seriously. It issued over forty publications aimed at the general public, and it solicited support from leading public officials; representatives of business, labor, and agriculture; and, of course, leaders in the public health, medical, and social welfare communities. The committee focused on health problems that could not be controlled by individual states. In a letter seeking support from health authorities, for example, Norton cited the following "facts" the committee had assembled:

> (a) *The facts*, that the Ohio River represents a thousand miles of typhoid fever, and the Hudson River a *cloaca maxima* from Albany to the sea; the prevalence of deadly infection among millions of our people, arising from the contamination of drinking water, and of ice, and the rapid increase of pollution of our rivers, the boundary lines between states, which only federal authority can control; or
>
> (b) *the facts*, that out of 80,000,000 of our people, 8,000,000 must perish from tuberculosis, the white scourge, which with proper regulation enforced by the federal power can be exterminated as completely as the once dreaded smallpox; and that the uniform enforcement of national health regulations in all states is absolutely imperative, because infected persons travel from state to state spreading the disease; or
>
> (c) *the facts*, that the bubonic plague has gained such a foothold in California that national aid was asked; that the plague has behind it a history of devastation more terrible than human words can portray, and should it once again gain a foothold in a crowded metropolis, and sporadic cases begin to develop, this disease will cost more in life and effort, than the

adequate appropriations for a great national organization of health operating over the period of a generation. Only by extending the national quarantine can other states be protected against laxity in the enforcement of health regulations by a single recalcitrant state; or

(d) *the facts*, that the milk-supplies of cities are often drawn from adjoining states over which state control is difficult to maintain; and that infant mortality varies directly with the purity of the milk supply; or

(e) *the facts*, that the public have no means of obtaining reliable health information, and the thousand questions which anxious fathers and mothers ask themselves go unanswered simply because there is no office at Washington equipped for the purpose. If strawberries wilt in New Jersey or lambs fall sick in Arizona the Department of Agriculture gives elaborate instructions as to what should be done. But two millions of human beings die each year—a large proportion, and literally because they cannot find out *how to live*.[28]

In 1909 the committee presented a report of its findings and recommendations to the National Conservation Commission. Written by committee president Irving Fisher, who was also a member of the National Conservation Commission, the document was entitled *A Report on National Vitality*. In the report, Fisher advocated the uniting of health units in many different government agencies under one head, who would be given cabinet rank. This should be done, he contended, so that "American vitality may reach its maximum development. . . . It is," he said, "both bad policy and bad economy to leave this work mainly to the weak and spasmodic efforts of charity, or to the philanthropy of physicians."[29]

Presidents Theodore Roosevelt and William Howard Taft endorsed the principles of the committee, although both were reluctant to increase the size of their cabinets. Roosevelt mentioned the need for "increasing interest on the part of the National Government" in public health in his seventh annual message, and more pointedly decried the "inadequacy of American public health legislation" in his eighth.[30] Taft recommended specifically the formation of a bureau of health in his first annual message.[31] A number of bills were introduced into Congress to establish the recommended department, or alternatively, a bureau of health. While the Committee of One Hundred had bowed to the view of President Taft that a cabinet-level department was unacceptable, they were confronted in February 1910 with a bill introduced by Oklahoma senator Robert L. Owen for just such a department.[32] Members of the committee, in a joint conference with representatives of the American Medical Association, decided not to risk alienating Taft by directly supporting the bill, but they agreed to endorse the "principle of a Department, although of course a Sub-Department or Bureau" might have to be accepted as a compromise.[33]

The reaction of the Public Health and Marine Hospital Service to the Owen bill was as strong as it had been to the National Board of Health legislation in the 1870s. Surgeon General Wyman, who had joined the Service three years before the battle over the National Board of Health began, was apparently as intent as his predecessors had been in directing the development of the Service into a national health department. He did not speak out directly against the Committee of One Hundred's proposals or against the Owen bill. In fact, he wrote to President Taft in 1909, "I have never opposed a Department of Health, with a Secretary in the Cabinet, for I have realized that development might in time make such a Department advisable."[34] His vision, of course, was that the Service should develop into such a department. Already he considered it to be both "de facto and de jure a public health service."[35]

What Wyman advocated at this time was an expansion of the Service on many fronts.[36] In the Hygienic Laboratory he wanted statute authority to investigate water pollution and noncontagious diseases. He hoped to rectify the imbalance in pay and perquisites between commissioned officers of the Service and those of the military. At the same time he hoped to make the Hygienic Laboratory Professors commissioned officers rather than civil servants.

In addition to these aims for the research effort of the Service, Wyman wanted the Hygienic Laboratory Advisory Board elevated to a Surgeon General's Advisory Board. The Hygienic Laboratory Advisory Board, although having met infrequently, had been warmly received by Service officials. The nongovernmental members, many of whom were leading health authorities in the nation, had encouraged research activities, and Wyman believed such men would be valuable as advisors on general public health problems. Another goal was a provision that would allow state, territorial, and municipal health officers to utilize the Hygienic Laboratory for graduate training in public health and to increase the number of meetings of the state and territorial health officers allowed each year. Moreover, Wyman wanted the federal government and not the states to pay the expenses of these meetings. Increased interaction, in addition to affording the latest methods to local health officers, would go a long way to bridge the states' rights chasm that had often hindered cooperation between federal and state authorities in the control of epidemic diseases. Wyman also wanted the Service authorized to publish information for the general public. The *Hygienic Laboratory Bulletin*, written for scientists, and the *Public Health Reports*, meant primarily for public health officials, were the only authorized publications of the Service. He also hoped for statutory authority to allow the Service to cooperate with other agencies of the government, a practice that had existed for some years without legislative mandate.

A series of bills embodying some or all of these plans was introduced between 1908 and 1912.[37] Congressman Mann of Illinois was the Service's chief congressional supporter in this effort. These bills, however, were put before Congress at the same time as the proposals endorsed by the Committee of One Hundred for a bureau or department of public health. The old antagonism between the Service and other public health leaders was kindled once again, more strongly than it had been at any time since the debates over the National Board of Health. John Shaw Billings, who had been the principal antagonist to the Service in that earlier battle, wrote to Irving Fisher that he had "no doubt" that the obstacles to the efforts of the Committee of One Hundred had been "mainly due to Surgeon General Wyman."[38] Fisher agreed and even discussed with committee members some way to have Wyman removed from office. Wyman, however, was cautious and temperate in his public statements, so his opposition could not find grounds for such action.

In 1910 some thirteen different bills relating to health, the Public Health and Marine Hospital Service, or the proposed national department of health were before Congress. In June 1910 and January 1911 the House Committee on Interstate and Foreign Commerce held lengthy hearings on all the measures.

A galaxy of public health figures spoke in favor of creating a department of health. Their number included prominent members of the Committee of One Hundred, the Surgeon General of the Navy, and a former Surgeon General of the Army. Their arguments were pure logic: such a department would promote economy and efficiency and would conserve a precious national resource. The inability of states to handle problems that crossed state lines was evident. Science had provided some keys and would surely provide more in the future to make disease control a simple matter of proper prevention.[39]

Bureaucrats such as Harvey W. Wiley, chief of the Bureau of Chemistry in the Department of Agriculture and leader of the pure food and drugs crusade, were more moderate in their endorsement of reforms needed. "I am not one of those who favor . . . the transferring of great bureaus," Wiley stated.[40] Coordination was his scheme for better efficiency, and he offered the example of the many chemical laboratories in the government in describing what should be done. Rather than consolidating all the chemical laboratories into one large facility,

Wiley proposed that the several laboratories be placed under a single administrator to achieve a "uniform method of doing work."[41]

Surprisingly strong opposition was voiced against the bills proposed both by the Committee of One Hundred and by the Service. John L. Bates, a former governor of Massachusetts, represented opposing views that had coalesced only three weeks before the hearings into a group calling itself the National League for Medical Freedom.[42] Claiming a membership of 69,800, including such notable people as Clara Barton of the Red Cross, the league specifically represented the interests of osteopaths, eclectics, homeopaths, Christian Scientists, antivivisectionists, and antivaccinationists. Irving Fisher alleged that the league, which was obviously well financed, was supported by patent medicine interests, who bitterly opposed legislation that might restrict their business further than the Pure Food and Drugs Act already had.[43] League representatives hotly denied such a connection.[44]

Bates concentrated his argument on the unconstitutionality of all the proposals. "Where," he asked, "in the . . . powers of Congress, can be found power to pass measures, as provided in the bills before you?"[45] Seeking the support of southern representatives who were traditionally strict constructionists on constitutional matters, Bates pointed out that the Constitution did not delegate to Congress the power to regulate health. H. L. Gordon, another spokesperson for the league, played on the fear of invasion of privacy by claiming that the measures would open "the door of every home in this country" to the Public Health and Marine Hospital Service and authorize them "to investigate any personal disease or personal sickness, wherever it may be."[46]

Representatives of irregular schools of medicine joined the chorus of opposing voices. They contended that the bills were the work of the American Medical Association, an organization they characterized as a "medical trust" that sought to destroy all competing schools of medicine.[47] Other speakers against the bills reviled orthodox medicine for its many failures past and present. They pointed to the debilitating heroic remedies of the past, such as bleeding and purging, and shuddered at existing problems such as anaphylactic shock and tetanus contracted from smallpox vaccinations. Children, an antivaccinationist stated graphically, should not be forced to have their "pure blood" contaminated with "calf pus."[48] Enactment of any of the bills, they argued, would allow orthodox medicine to make such treatments mandatory.

Proponents of the bills as well as members of the National League for Medical Freedom bombarded members of Congress with letters and telegrams.[49] The league also took out large advertisements in the *Washington Herald* and the *Washington Post*.[50] When the smoke had cleared, Congress responded predictably to such a highly contested issue: it did not act.

Nothing at all might have resulted from these debates had not Walter Wyman died suddenly in November 1911 in a diabetic coma. His successor was Rupert Blue, an officer who had won an international reputation by successfully suppressing bubonic plague in California. Blue and his superior, Secretary of the Treasury Franklin MacVeagh, pressed strongly for enactment of scaled-down legislation suggested by Wyman. Responding perhaps out of respect for the dead Surgeon General, and probably out of a desire to do something not wracked with controversy to pacify health reformers, Congress passed the measure, which was introduced by Congressman Mann. It was signed by President Taft on August 14, 1912.[51]

The brief 1912 act shortened the name of the Service to "Public Health Service," and provided for three of the many reforms proposed by Wyman. The change in name acknowledged that public health was indeed the Service's main concern, conferring a status that many felt was long overdue. The act authorized the publication of information "for the use of the public," raised the pay of commissioned officers, and granted the Service the right to "investigate the diseases of man and conditions influencing the propagation and spread thereof, including sanitation and sewage and the pollution either directly or indirectly of the navigable streams and lakes of the United States." The Service was able, with this law, to go forward with its research into noncontagious diseases and to conduct pioneering studies on water pollution.

The Division of Chemistry, for example, under the leadership of Earle B. Phelps, began studies of water pollution and of the biochemistry of sewage and industrial wastes.[52] Phelps and his staff put forth the "original formulation of the basic law of the biochemical oxygen-demand reaction and its temperature coefficient."[53] Their formulations of this and the well known "oxygen-sag" curve were classics in the field, assisting work on sewage and on pollution of rivers and other bodies of water.[54] Joseph Goldberger, moreover, was able under this law to continue his investigations of pellagra. Congress even authorized special appropriations for this work from 1913 to 1921.[55] The new law provided the Laboratory with increased independence from the more routine activities of the Service and enhanced its position. "As the scientific work of the Service proceeds," remarked Assistant Surgeon General John Kerr, director of the Division of Scientific Research, in his section of the Service's 1915 annual report, the importance of the Hygienic Laboratory "becomes more and more apparent. It is safe to say that the results obtained from one line of study alone have been of many times greater value than the entire appropriation for studies of public health matters for the year."[56]

The 1912 law failed, however, to address the other problems Wyman had hoped to solve. The position of the Hygienic Laboratory Professors was not improved. Reid Hunt, director of the Division of Pharmacology, was quickly lured away by Harvard Medical School, and E. C. Franklin, Earle Phelps's predecessor as the director of the Division of Chemistry, moved to Stanford University. The Hygienic Laboratory Advisory Board did not become a national public health advisory body. States continued to bear the cost of the annual meeting of their health officers with the Surgeon General. The Service cooperated with other departments of government from time to time, but with no statutory authority to do so. Moreover, in addition to not reducing the large number of health agencies scattered throughout the federal bureaucracy, a new bureau was created. In 1912 the Children's Bureau was established to address the problems of child labor, health, and education. This agency, supported strongly by Progressive reformers, had been offered to Surgeon General Wyman before his death as a possible new division in the Service. Wyman, a bachelor, "refused to complicate his life with the importunities of a group of sentimental women who were interested solely in the welfare of mothers and infants."[57] The Children's Bureau was placed in the Labor Department and developed its own health program.

After the enactment of the 1912 law, the efforts of the Committee of One Hundred dwindled. Senator Owen continued to reintroduce his bill, and he received support from Louisiana senator Joseph E. Ransdell, chairman of the Senate Committee on Public Health and National Quarantine. Some interest was also expressed by Surgeon General Blue, who proposed an alternative bill that would have transferred other health bureaus into the Public Health Service and created an assistant secretary of health in the Treasury Department.[58] With the advent of World War I, however, the interest of Congress was directed elsewhere, and no action was taken on these proposals.

The Great War placed new demands on the Public Health Service and its leader, Rupert Blue.[59] Born in North Carolina, Blue received his M.D. from the University of Maryland in 1892. In his early career with the Service, he was stationed at a variety of ports for duty in hospital and quarantine work. In 1903 and 1907 Blue was in charge of operations to control bubonic plague in San Francisco. He developed extensive rat extermination drives that dramatically halted the epidemic and demonstrated that plague was carried by fleas on rats rather than by human carriers.[60] This work catapulted him to Surgeon General in 1912 over the heads of more seasoned officers. The monthly *Medical Times* in New York hailed his appointment, saying that President Taft had "forgot the bugbear of precedence and nominated the best man."[61]

A quiet man, Blue was a conscientious scientist. He seemed, however, to lack the political intuition that characterized his predecessor. Elected to the presidency of the American Medical Association in 1916—the first and last Surgeon General of the Public Health Service to be so honored—Blue gave his presidential address in 1917 at a time when it was becoming clear the United States would become involved in the World War. He proposed to organize a committee to study how the facilities of the American Medical Association could be used in preparing for war.[62]

The activities of the Service and its Hygienic Laboratory were likewise redirected to meet wartime needs. Blue was prepared to set up health service facilities around training camps, but he found that no federal funds existed for such purposes.[63] The American Red Cross assumed the financial burden for creating a Bureau of Sanitary Services. In November 1917 frustrated commissioned officers petitioned the Surgeon General to be assigned to the military for the duration of the war.[64] Treasury Secretary William McAdoo moved swiftly to halt this movement, and shortly thereafter Congress increased the funds available to the Service for controlling epidemics around military installations.[65] To meet a need for increased personnel, moreover, Surgeon General Blue "directed the preparation of a bill" to create a Reserve Officer Corps in the Service.[66] The legislation was stalled in Congress until October 1918 and became law only after the period of greatest need had passed.[67]

In 1918 an additional $1 million was appropriated for the Service in an attempt to "combat and suppress 'Spanish influenza,'" the disease that appeared first in Spain but rapidly spread to pandemic proportions.[68] Regrettably, neither the Service nor local physicians could do much to halt the disease. Medical research had made little headway against the influenza virus.[69] The Service utilized the appropriated monies to employ additional physicians, nurses, and nurses' aids to travel, if necessary, to afflicted areas and offer assistance to overtaxed local personnel. Hygienic Laboratory physicians, who generally had not practiced medicine during their research careers, were also called upon to treat government workers in temporary hospitals set up in

Washington.[70] The severity of the disease, which was not even an internationally reportable illness before the pandemic, pointed up the need for research into its cause and treatment as well as close monitoring of its incidence.

Hygienic Laboratory research during the war was "related almost entirely to health problems arising out of the war."[71] Such problems were many, and they demanded quick solutions. The largest effort undertaken was the grouping of organisms isolated from cases of epidemic meningitis. Laboratory director George McCoy and bacteriologist Ida Bengtson also demonstrated the presence of tetanus organisms on bone points commonly used to scarify the skin in smallpox vaccinations. This work led to the abandonment of bone points in the administration of vaccinations to military personnel during the war. Laboratory personnel identified shaving brushes used by troops as the source of some cases of tetanus and anthrax. Tetanus antitoxin was supplied to the British Army before the United States entered the war, and an antityphoid vaccine developed in the Laboratory protected the troops of nations on both sides of the conflict. John McMullen's work on trachoma was utilized to treat recruits suffering from that eye disease rather than rejecting them automatically. Special studies on industrial fatigue were accomplished. The Laboratory was also charged with controlling the distribution of pathogenic organisms used in medical research. Careful regulation was necessary, in order that the germs not fall into the hands of ill-intentioned persons.[72]

Two wartime measures affecting the Service served as precedents for later legislative proposals. President Woodrow Wilson issued an executive order in July 1918 that placed "all sanitary or public health activities carried on by any executive" agency under the supervision of the secretary of the Treasury. Wilson's reasons were "to avoid confusion in policies, duplication of effort, and to bring about more effective results."[73] The order remained in effect only until hostilities ceased, but it was cited as a rationale for later efforts to achieve a similar organization during peacetime. A second measure, enacted by Congress, established an Interdepartmental Social Hygiene Board to investigate the cause of and find methods to control venereal disease, a problem that plagued the military during the war.[74] This act created a Division of Venereal Diseases in the Public Health Service with an appropriation of $200,000. It also set aside $100,000 to be awarded as grants to university and other nongovernmental scientists for work on venereal diseases and $300,000 for sociological and psychological research leading to better educational measures. Not since the National Board of Health had awarded grants for the investigation of yellow fever in the 1880s had the federal government allocated funds for biomedical research.[75] This provision would also serve as a precedent for future grants outside the government.

At the end of World War I, Surgeon General Blue proposed a comprehensive plan for national and international health.[76] The program included broad powers for federal, state, and local public health officers. Blue suggested, for example, the establishment of clinics for sick children, minimum standards of permissible pollution in water supplies, universal pasteurization of milk, and the free distribution of arsphenamine to combat syphilis. He was vague about how the cost for these programs would be apportioned, and he included a number of recommendations, such as universal pasteurization, that were strongly opposed by many people. His proposals were not enacted, because his term as Surgeon General ended in 1920, and Secretary of the Treasury Carter Glass was determined to consider only a fellow Virginian for the post.[77] When Blue stepped down as Surgeon General, the Public Health Service was significantly larger than when he took office, primarily because of expansion during World War I. The Service had been assigned to assist the War Risk Insurance Bureau by providing medical care for veterans, an enormous expansion over its previous commitment to merchant seamen.[78] Blue had experienced great difficulties in obtaining funds and additional personnel quickly, however, and little progress had been made in improving the status or salaries of commissioned officers and the nonmedical scientific staff. These groups felt that Service personnel were in a "dormant" period under Blue.[79] It is possible to speculate that in choosing the best scientist for Surgeon General, President Taft might have overlooked a better administrator.

The first two decades of the twentieth century were a time in which the Hygienic Laboratory began to develop as a research center with considerable independence. Under the leadership of Milton Rosenau, John Anderson, and George McCoy, it gained an international reputation for work of the highest quality. Although its work focused on practical problems in accordance with scientific and public consensus regarding the appropriate work of government laboratories, researchers were able under the provisions of the 1912 act to expand their investigations into new fields such as nutritional diseases. It was not only the Laboratory's research that contributed to its permanence in the federal bureaucracy; a large part of its legitimacy as a government agency obtained from the efficient manner in which it enforced the Biologics Control Act of 1902. The demands of World War I further contributed to the conviction that such a research arm of the Public Health Service was valuable to the government. As the United States settled into the postwar "normalcy" period, Assistant Surgeon General J. W. Schereschewsky, then the Service's director of the Scientific Research Division, observed that the war had "emphasized the importance of public health work." The combined effect of the 1918 influenza epidemic and the finding that one-third of the men of military age were unfit for duty, he said, was evidence of "a crying need that more attention be paid by the Federal Government to the problems of public health."[80] Specifically, he looked forward to the new decade as one in which the Laboratory could continue "on a much larger scale" the research begun in the opening decades of the twentieth century.

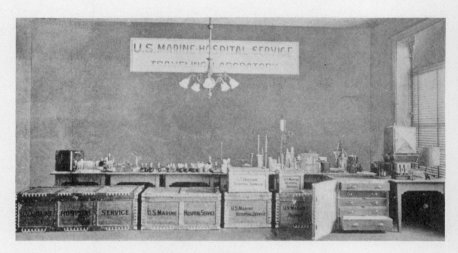

To provide Marine Hospital Service officers stationed in remote locations at the turn of the century with necessary tools for making bacteriological diagnoses of infectious diseases, the Hygienic Laboratory developed this portable laboratory. Its contents included a microscope, incubator, sterilizer, media, stains, and some glassware. Photograph from the *Annual Report of the Supervising Surgeon of the Marine Hospital Service, 1900.*

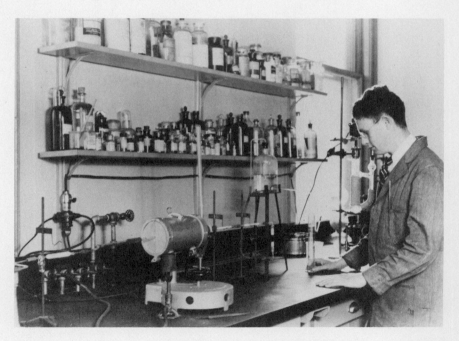

The relative simplicity of the portable laboratory is contrasted with the wide variety of equipment available by the 1930s, some of which is shown being used by a laboratory assistant. Photograph courtesy of the National Library of Medicine.

Charles Wardell Stiles, first director of the Hygienic Laboratory's Division of Zoology, endured some abuse for mentioning in public the problem of human waste disposal. Undaunted, he designed in 1910 an inexpensive sanitary privy, the merits of which were advocated in the handbill shown in this photograph. Both photographs courtesy of the National Library of Medicine.

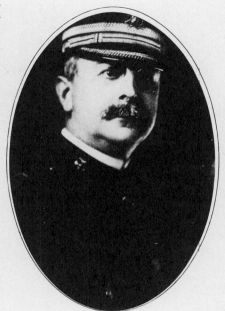

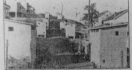

(To Be Tacked Inside of the Privy and NOT Torn Down.)

Sanitary Privies Are Cheaper Than Coffins

For Health's Sake let's keep this Privy CLEAN. Bad privies (and no privies at all) are our greatest cause of Disease. Clean people or families will help us keep this place clean. It should be kept as clean as the house because it spreads more diseases.

The User Must Keep It Clean Inside. Wash the Seat Occasionally

How to Keep a Safe Privy:

1. *Have the back perfectly screened against flies and animals.*
2. *Have a hinged door over the seat and keep it CLOSED when not in use.*
3. *Have a bucket beneath to catch the Excreta.*
4. *VENTILATE THE VAULT.*
5. *See that the privy is kept clean inside and out, or take the blame on yourself if some member of your family dies of Typhoid Fever.*

Some of the Diseases Spread by Filthy Privies:

Typhoid Fever, Bowel Troubles of Children, Dysenteries, Hookworms, Cholera, some Tuberculosis. The Flies that You See in the Privy Will Soon Be in the Dining Room.

Walker County Board of Health

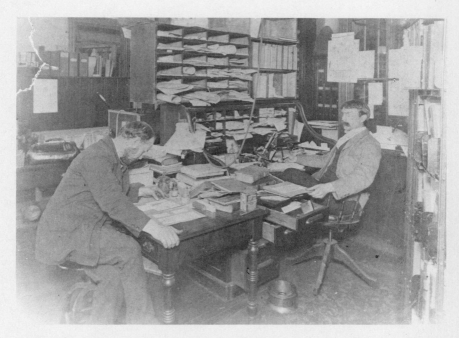

Charles Wardell Stiles and Albert Hassall, who together produced the monumental *Index-Catalog of Medical and Veterinary Zoology*, collaborating in Stiles's office. Photograph courtesy of the National Library of Medicine.

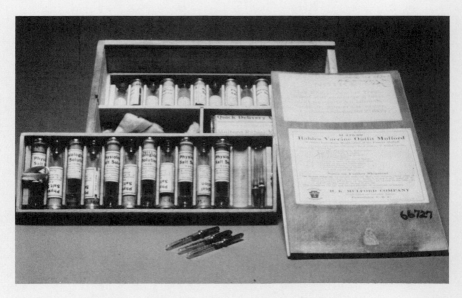

Under the provisions of the Biologics Control Act of 1902, the Hygienic Laboratory became the agency charged with enforcing purity and potency requirements for vaccines, sera, and antitoxins produced by commercial firms. This rabies vaccine outfit produced by the H. K. Mulford Company, with its twenty-one increasingly virulent doses, could be used by physicians with confidence that its contents were not contaminated with, for example, lethal tetanus organisms. Photograph courtesy of the National Museum of American History, Smithsonian Institution.

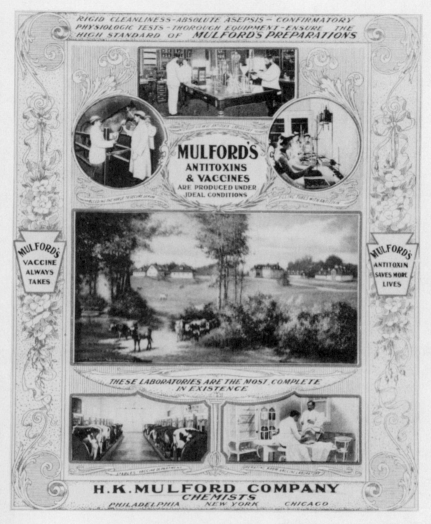

Production of vaccines and antitoxins, pictured in this 1900 catolog cover, was a meticulous process. The 1902 Biologics Control Act authorized the Hygienic Laboratory to inspect firms and grant licenses to those that met rigorous standards of cleanliness. Photograph courtesy of the National Museum of American History, Smithsonian Institution.

In 1912 Congress broadened the authority of
the Hygienic Laboratory, authorizing it to investigate not only infectious and contagious diseases but nutritional diseases as well. Under
this expanded mandate, Joseph Goldberger conducted brilliant epidemiological studies that linked
pellagra, a scourge of the poor in the South, to
their deficient diet. Photograph courtesy of the
National Library of Medicine.

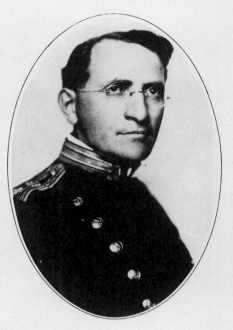

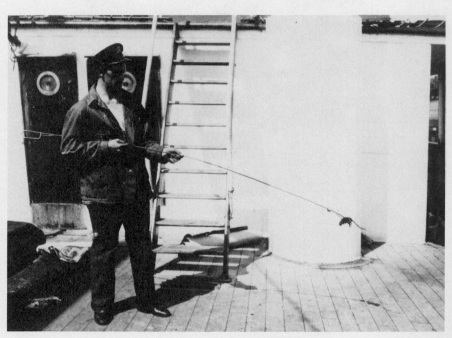

Bubonic plague, one of the most feared epidemic diseases, was a focus of investigations and practical
control efforts by the Hygienic Laboratory during its periodic visitations in the United States. An
unidentified seaman demonstrates in this photograph one safe way to handle a rat potentially harboring
plague-infected fleas. Photograph courtesy of the National Library of Medicine.

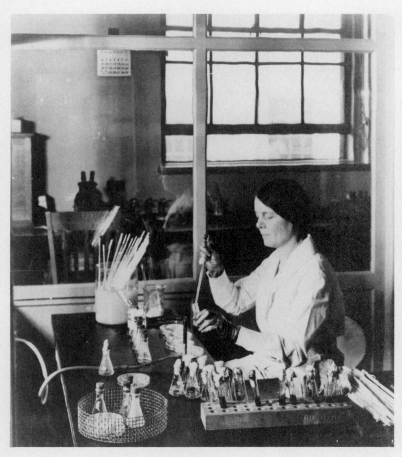

In 1916 Ida A. Bengtson became the first woman to hold a professional position in the Hygienic Laboratory. She subsequently earned high regard for studies of bacterial toxins, trachoma, and rickettsial diseases. For the women who followed her, wrote a colleague, "it was well . . . that the pioneer woman . . . was filling her position so ably." Photograph courtesy of the National Library of Medicine.

THREE

Alliance with the National Health Movement

It is about time that a practical plan for the centralization of federal health work, now widely scattered and uncoordinated, is proposed by a national organization with knowledge enough to understand the matter and energy enough to attempt to get it adopted.

James A. Tobey, 1924

The battles fought by public health leaders to establish a national department of health helped to solidify these individuals into what Charles-Edward Amory Winslow called the "national health movement."[1] This movement was concerned with many facets of public health, including the expansion of personal hygiene through public education, the promotion of health insurance schemes so that all citizens could receive medical care, and the extension of preventive medicine through health departments and visiting nurses. In some of these efforts the movement ran afoul of the American Medical Association (AMA), which maintained that therapy was the exclusive right of physicians and opposed, by 1920, national health insurance plans.[2] Such differences encouraged public health leaders to attempt to define a role for public health distinct from that of physicians.[3] In this effort the concept of a national public health department remained one policy priority. By the 1920s, however, the national health movement had virtually abandoned crusades such as that of the Committee of One Hundred. Instead, it sought to ally itself with the Public Health Service in order to achieve its ends through the existing bureaucracy. Expressed in the popular political terms of New Era politics, this purpose was to achieve better coordination and efficiency in government health agencies through consolidation of bureaus wherever possible. Such an alliance was not rejected by the Service, as it might have been in an earlier period, because the proposals of the national health movement did not threaten the Service's hegemony within the federal establishment. Furthermore, leaders of the Service had been frustrated in achieving several internal reforms that were felt to be essential, and cooperation with a strong health lobby such as the national health movement increased the possibility that Service goals might be achieved.

Many of the difficulties faced by the Service in advancing its legislative program were related to other New Era schemes to promote efficiency and ferret out duplication and waste in government. Early in his administration, President Warren G. Harding had created a Bureau of the Budget in order to provide a coherent economic program for the nation instead of relying on the piecemeal appropriations previously made by Congress. Charles G. Dawes was named first director of the bureau in 1921; he resigned the following year after establishing the bureau's policies and was succeeded by Herbert Mayhew Lord, a retired brigadier general of the Army who had been director of finance for the Army during World War I.[4]

For the aspirations of the Public Health Service in the 1920s, Lord's appointment as Budget director had significant consequences. He subscribed to a philosophy of rigid economy in government, but his fiscal conservatism was sometimes applied selectively. He was more inclined to approve appropriations increases for the military services than for civilian agencies such as the Public Health Service because, like many conservative congressmen, he was suspicious of the Service's commission system for officers, believing that employees of a civilian agency should not be assigned ranks as military physicians were.[5] Because Lord was also a Christian Scientist, he had little personal interest in the expansion of public health or of medical research programs.[6] Since the Budget Bureau had to approve any bill that carried an appropriation, however, Lord was an obstacle that had to be overcome before health legislation could be enacted.

The years 1918 through 1920 had been tumultuous for the Public Health Service. Demands made on it by wartime necessity and the influenza pandemic of 1918 had not been relieved before Congress added new responsibilities when it created the War Risk Insurance Bureau in 1919 to care for veterans of World War I. The new bureau had no existing staff or facilities, so Congress assigned the medical care of veterans to the Public Health Service but provided that the Service would function as an agency of the War Risk Insurance Bureau in performing these duties. This peculiar status prevented the Service from developing long-term policies for this massive undertaking and caused significant stress internally over matters of personnel.[7] Additional Service officers, sanitary engineers, dentists, pharmacists, and nurses were all needed, but pay for Service officers was low and Civil Service compensation for the other groups was penurious. When the inflation of the postwar period further eroded the earning capacity of these groups, the Service faced a crisis in acquiring and maintaining quality professionals for all of its varied activities.

To deal with these problems, the Service had sponsored several bills in the early 1920s. One would have authorized the president to transfer some dentists, sanitary engineers, and scientists from the Reserve Corps of the Service to the Commissioned Corps and would have permitted the Service to establish a nurse corps.[8] This bill was first introduced in 1921 and in modified form again in 1924. Another series of bills in the same years would have authorized the commissioning of sanitary engineers.[9] These bills were thwarted by General Lord in the Budget Bureau and by his congressional sympathizers.

Because of these difficulties, leaders of the Service were amenable to several proposals for reorganizing the federal bureaucracy that would remove the medical care of veterans from their agency or at least clarify their position in relationship to the War Risk Insurance Bureau. One of these proposals was initiated by President Harding in response to pressure from veterans' groups for better coordination of veterans' services. Harding appointed Charles Sawyer, a homeopath from Ohio who was the White House physician, to survey existing agencies that dealt with the health, education, and welfare of veterans.[10] Sawyer's work led to the consolidation of the War Risk Insurance Bureau, the Federal Board for Vocational Education, and the medical services that had been provided by the Public Health Service into a central Veterans' Bureau.[11] The transfer of facilities and staff out of the Service and into the new bureau relieved some pressure on the Public Health Service. Until 1924, however, it continued to assign some personnel to the Veterans' Bureau and to be responsible for the care of veterans outside the continental limits of the United States.[12]

At the same time that Sawyer's investigation was underway, Congress was also considering reorganization schemes that went beyond the creation of one new bureau. In 1920, before Harding had been inaugurated, Congress had passed a joint resolution establishing a committee to study and recommend all necessary changes in administrative departments to achieve more coordination and efficiency.[13] Composed of three members of each house of Congress, the committee was headed by Utah senator Reed Smoot and Nebraska congressman C. F. Reavis.[14] In 1922 the Smoot-Reavis committee considered a proposal to create a new department of education and public welfare that would consolidate the new Veterans' Bureau with the Public Health Service, other federal health agencies, and an assortment of educational and welfare agencies. The Public Health Service had not strongly objected to other proposals for coordination of agencies, but it balked at the Smoot-Reavis scheme.[15] Leaders of the Service believed that the Veterans' Bureau was so large that it would overshadow all other agencies in a combined department.

Another reason that the Service was reluctant to accept the recommendations of the Smoot-Reavis committee was a perception that Senator Smoot was no friend of public health. Early in 1921, for example, Smoot had attacked the Service in the Senate during debate on an appropriations bill providing for additional personnel. He charged that the Surgeon General, "while himself an honest and capable man, was surrounded by men with no respect for Congress and no mercy on the Treasury."[16] A Mormon and an avowed fiscal conservative, Smoot was backed by his junior colleague from Utah, William King, who further alleged that the Service was trying to "Russianize this republic," determined to "go into the states, and to discharge the duties and responsibilities which belong to the citizens and to local communities."[17] Smoot and King, like Budget director Lord, opposed any change that would bring the civilian Public Health Service status more nearly in line with that of the military.

The new Surgeon General of the Public Health Service who was faced with these formidable reorganization plans was Hugh Smith Cumming. Born in 1869 in Hampton, Virginia, Cumming received his M.D. from the University of Virginia in 1892.[18] After joining the Service, he was assigned to quarantine work at Ellis Island and in San Francisco and Japan. He also participated in the pollution studies of navigable streams authorized by the 1912 act.[19] After World War I Cumming was assigned to the sanitary commission that surveyed European health conditions. He was, in fact, representing the Service at official international meetings when word arrived of his nomination to be Surgeon General.[20]

A tall, thin man of patrician bearing, Cumming had many acquaintances and apparently enjoyed the political maneuvering required of a successful Surgeon General. In a profile of Cumming prepared by the *New York Times* in 1928, he was described as "knowing virtually everyone in Washington" and having friends "throughout the United States and abroad."[21] Cumming's views on the function of the Public Health Service were inclined to reflect the states' rights conservatism of his native South. He believed that "the local community and the State" had a "fundamental responsibility in health matters," and he had "little sympathy for those who would transfer this responsibility to Washington."[22] Cumming, then, was hardly inclined to ride roughshod over the prerogatives of the states in health matters as Senators Smoot and King suggested.

The initial proposal of the Smoot-Reavis committee for a department of education and welfare was never enacted. Cumming and the heads of other bureaus opposed the move, and the committee's recommendation was put aside when President Harding died in August 1923.[23] With the backing of the new administration of Calvin Coolidge, however, in early 1925 the committee's bill for the establishment of what was then designated a department of education and relief was taken up by Congress. Reed Smoot sponsored the proposal in the Senate and Michigan congressman Carl Mapes introduced the bill in the House.

The Public Health Service and the American Public Health Association strongly opposed the Smoot-Mapes bill because the Veterans' Bureau was included in the proposed department. This large bureau, an editorial in the *American Journal of Public Health* observed, would constitute "about ninety percent of the department" and with the Bureau of Pensions "would completely overshadow both education and public health."[24] Under another provision described as "drastic and dangerous" in this editorial, the director of the proposed department could abolish any office or change the organizational structure of the department at will. Such power, another observer commented, would have the effect of "throwing the whole personnel at the mercy of any political change."[25] Cumming contacted his many friends in the medical profession about the bill, asking for their support in opposing it. "When you consider," Cumming wrote to urologist Hugh H. Young at Johns Hopkins, that "the dominant factors are now General Lord, a Christian Scientist, and Smoot, a Mormon who has always been opposed to public health, you can see the danger in this proposition."[26] The response of these physicians was overwhelmingly negative toward the bill, and it was defeated.

These administrative problems fought by the leadership of the Public Health Service had some impact on the Hygienic Laboratory, especially in the areas of research budgets and personnel. The research work of the Laboratory was conducted under an annual maintenance appropriation supplemented by specific appropriations for special projects. The latter, which included pellagra investigations and work on venereal disease, were always subject to drastic cutting according to political priorities. In 1919, for example, Congress first appropriated $200,000 for work on venereal diseases, increased it to $400,000 in 1923, but cut it severely in 1926 to $75,000. Venereal disease had not been cured or controlled by that time, but it was no longer the important political concern it had been in World War I. Joseph Goldberger's investigations of pellagra were also phased out by 1924, although in this case the dietary nature of the disease had been established and further research centered on identifying the "pellagra preventative factor" in foods.

The routine and ongoing work of the Laboratory, therefore, was conducted under the yearly maintenance appropriation. From 1907, when records on this item began to be recorded separately in the Service's annual report, the maintenance appropriation had risen slowly, in a stepwise manner.[27] In 1907 the amount was $15,000; it increased to $20,000 in 1914 and stayed level until the postwar inflation of 1919 when it jumped to $27,000. In the early 1920s it increased rapidly: in 1920 to $36,000; in 1921 to $45,000; and in 1922 it peaked at $50,000. The stringent economy measures of the Coolidge administration caused a rapid contraction. By 1926, the maintenance appropriation was down to $43,000, where it stayed until 1931. When adjusted for economic fluctuations, these figures show that the Service suffered during the inflation of World War I, recovered as the war ended, and felt the pinch of the cutbacks of the 1920s.[28]

In this same period the staff of the Laboratory had increased significantly, growing from 55 in 1909 to 117 in 1925.[29] More importantly, the scientific staff of the Laboratory had more than tripled in this period, from 15 to 46. As the 1920s began, the interests of Hygienic Laboratory scientists had expanded considerably from the early twentieth-century focus on infectious diseases. In the 1921 annual report, the director of the Division of Scientific Research observed that the "need is urgent to extend research work of the Federal Government into the causes and prevention of the diseases of man."[30] Specifically, director J. W. Schereschewsky pointed to the problems "of the so-called degenerative diseases, such as organic disease of the heart and other lesions of the cardio-vascular system, cancer, and kidney disease."[31] The following year, he reemphasized this larger focus by calling for the addition of a division of physiology to the Hygienic Laboratory.[32] Researchers in the Service, like their counterparts in universities and medical schools, wanted to enlarge their scope to include the less dramatic but more deadly and disabling chronic problems. As one step in this direction, Schereschewsky made arrangements in August 1922 with Milton J. Rosenau, former director of the Hygienic Laboratory and then chairman of the Department of Preventive Medicine and Hygiene at Harvard Medical School, for the Service to utilize the Harvard laboratories for a field investigation of cancer and other malignant growths.[33] This arrangement was informal, for existing law made no provision for such sharing of facilities.

Accompanying this expansion of interest was a desire to pursue lines of research in the Hygienic Laboratory that would be described as basic rather than applied. Laboratory Director George W. McCoy noted cautiously in 1922 that such a policy had been adopted "so far as practicable" and that "gratifying results" had been achieved.[34] The

most obvious example of such work was that of William Mansfield
Clark, who became the director of the Division of Chemistry in the
Hygienic Laboratory in 1920.[35] When he arrived at the Laboratory
from his previous post with the Dairy Division of the Department of
Agriculture, Clark had just published a book that was to become a
classic on the subject of acid-base equilibria, *The Determination of
Hydrogen Ions.*[36] During his seven-year tenure at the Hygienic Laboratory, Clark turned to the study of oxidation-reduction potentials.
Another distinguished biochemist remarked in 1965 about this work:
"His first ten papers of the series *Studies on Oxidation-Reduction*,
published between 1923 and 1926, stand today as milestones in the
theory, measurement, and interpretation of oxidation-reduction as applied to organic systems."[37]

While Clark's work was hailed as a "milestone" and described as
classic, it was much less clear that it fit conveniently into the legislated
mission of the Hygienic Laboratory to investigate the diseases of man.
As the hookworm and pellagra studies raised questions in the first
decade of the century about how they could be justified as "infectious
and contagious diseases," so basic research strained the limits of
existing law that referred only to disease-oriented research. Leaders
of the Service, who believed that fundamental research was an essential part of their work, were willing to interpret the law broadly,
as McCoy did. Others believed that a more definite statement was
needed to protect basic research as a legitimate line of inquiry for
federal medical research, but this reasoning is the subject of a later
chapter.

By 1925 the Service and its Hygienic Laboratory had expanded
considerably since the 1902 and 1912 acts that defined federal policy
for public health and medical research. Many Service leaders believed
that changes were needed, but few believed that Service proposals
would be welcomed by Budget director Lord or by conservative congressmen. A way out of this frustrating situation was presented in
1926 when some members of the national health movement launched
a new campaign to consolidate federal health agencies, a New Era
version of the old national department of health proposal.

The originators of this scheme were leaders of the National Health
Council, a nongovernmental organization composed of volunteer health
agencies. The council was in many ways an outgrowth of the former
Committee of One Hundred. In 1913, after their drive to consolidate
federal health activities had failed, some members of the committee,
who were also members of the American Medical Association, turned
their energies to the coordination of nongovernmental agencies. In
April of that year a conference of thirty-nine health agencies was held

at the request of the Council on Health and Public Instruction of the AMA, and Professor Selskar M. Gunn of the Massachusetts Institute of Technology was appointed to make a study of problems relating to the coordination of these agencies.[38] In 1915 Gunn reported that there were twenty-four national organizations with a major interest in health. World War I interrupted further plans at that time, but after the war, the American Public Health Association called another conference on the subject, which resulted in another study by Donald B. Armstrong of the Metropolitan Life Insurance Company.

The National Health Council was the result of these years of study. It began to function January 1, 1921, with Livingston Farrand, a former member of the Committee of One Hundred and representative of the American Red Cross, as chairman. Armstrong was named executive officer. The council was composed of representatives of many national health organizations, including the American Heart Association, the American Public Health Association (APHA), the National Organization for Public Health Nursing, and the American Society for the Control of Cancer.[39] Advisory members were representatives of the Children's Bureau and the Public Health Service. Many member organizations transferred their headquarters to a common building in New York City where they could share office supplies and other resources.

Although the council was an alliance of many health organizations, the Metropolitan Life Insurance Company figured prominently in its leadership. Lee K. Frankel, a vice-president of Metropolitan Life and also a former member of the Committee of One Hundred, was vice-chairman of the council in 1921 and 1922 and chairman in 1923 and 1924.[40] Donald B. Armstrong, executive officer of the council from 1921 through 1923, was also a Metropolitan employee. A physician trained in public health, Armstrong had directed the 1916 town health demonstration project in Framingham, Massachusetts, that was co-sponsored by Metropolitan Life and the National Tuberculosis Association.[41]

Metropolitan Life had been active in preventive medicine since 1909.[42] Frankel, who at that time directed the Welfare Division of the company, inaugurated a visiting nurse program for the company's largely industrial policyholders.[43] In 1913, moreover, Frankel and Irving Fisher, with Eugene Lyman Fisk, medical director of the Provident Savings Life Association, formed the Life Extension Institute. For "an annual fee of $20, an individual would receive a health examination and be able to participate in all educational activities of the Institute."[44] In 1914 Metropolitan Life arranged for its policyholders to receive free examinations at the institute. This concerted public health campaign by the life insurance company had dramatic results. Within nine years, the mortality rate among policyholders declined 20 percent.[45] Preventive medicine plainly was profitable for Metropolitan Life. As leaders of the National Health Council, Frankel and Armstrong could speak with some authority about the benefits of coordinated preventive medicine campaigns.

The council engaged in a variety of activities. It prepared a study of voluntary health work in "a number of states," participated in a national campaign for the promotion of health examinations—an extension of the successful Metropolitan Life program—cooperated in developing a Hall of Health in the Smithsonian Institution, maintained a library of publications on health subjects, and edited a National Health Series published by Funk and Wagnalls. It issued biweekly reports on pending national health legislation and prepared reports on the health activities of federal bureaus.[46] These latter two activities were the responsibility of the council's Washington, D.C., representative, who in 1921 and 1922 was James Alner Tobey.

Tobey was a young man with wide-ranging interests. He had obtained a degree in sanitary engineering from the Massachusetts Institute of Technology in 1916, had been "a health officer in New Jersey, a scientific assistant in the Public Health Service," and a staff member of the American Red Cross.[47] After serving as the National Health Council's representative in Washington, D.C., for two years, Tobey became administrative secretary to the council in 1923. "While engaged in these activities," he "had obtained a master's degree from American University, a law degree from Southeastern, and was working toward his doctor's degree in public health, which he would obtain from M.I.T. in 1927."[48]

The National Health Council was closely allied with the leadership of the American Public Health Association. Throughout the 1920s, Tobey wrote a monthly column on public health law and legislation for the association's *Journal*. He had followed the activities of the Smoot-Reavis committee from the beginning, observing optimistically in 1921 that the proposed reorganization was "an opportunity such as has never before been presented."[49] When the final plan was presented in 1924, however, its attention to health matters was, in Tobey's opinion, incomplete. "It is about time," he stated in his July 1924 column, "that a practical plan for the centralization of federal health work, now widely scattered and uncoordinated, is proposed by a national organization with knowledge enough to understand the matter and energy enough to attempt to get it adopted. The National Health Council is undoubtedly the agency to do this."[50]

Later that year, at a dinner presided over by Livingston Farrand, a plan for centralization of health activities in the federal government was discussed by other leaders of the American Public Health Association.[51] They took the case to the association's annual meeting in St. Louis in October 1925 and won a resolution calling for "more effective centralization of federal health work under the direction of a competent, trained official who shall have the rank at least of an Assistant Secretary."[52] The resolution also stipulated that the centralized department contain "as many as practical of the bureaus engaged in public health and preventive medicine" with the specific exclusion of the Veterans' Bureau, and it authorized the president of the APHA to appoint a committee "to bring these resolutions and sentiments to the attention of President Coolidge and appropriate committees of Congress, and to cooperate with other groups who are studying and promoting federal health correlation."[53] The committee appointed was chaired by Lee K. Frankel, chairman of the National Health Council, and included Haven Emerson, professor of public health at Columbia University; Milton J. Rosenau, professor of preventive medicine and hygiene at Harvard University; William F. Snow, director of the American Social Hygiene Association; Linsly R. Williams, managing director of the National Tuberculosis Association; Charles-Edward Amory Winslow, professor of public health at Yale University, and James A. Tobey.

The National Health Council had already begun working on the federal health reorganization plan before this APHA Commission was formed. Tobey was authorized to publish a study of the health agencies of the federal government in which he would show how the work overlapped.[54] Financial support for the undertaking was obtained, not surprisingly, from the Metropolitan Life Insurance Company. Tobey did the work as a staff member of the Institute for Government Research, an association sponsored by Robert S. Brookings, which later merged with the Brookings Institution. In 1926 the institute published the results of Tobey's research as a book entitled *The National Government and Public Health*.

Tobey's book traced the historical development of public health in the federal government, analyzed the existing federal health activities in various bureaus, and proposed improved correlation of these activities. Tobey's legal training had served him well. The book was well researched from constitutional, statutory, administrative, and judicial documents on public health. Tobey found that of the approximately one hundred agencies in the federal government, more than forty were involved in public health in some capacity. In 1926 there were, he said, "seven distinct bureaus or divisions located in five different executive departments, which carry on public health work of such importance as to justify its classification as the major activity of the particular bureau or division."[55]

The Departments of War, the Interior, Labor, and Agriculture had the largest involvement outside of the Public Health Service. The Children's Bureau of the Labor Department, headed by the energetic Grace Abbott, was involved in a broad program of maternal and child care with monies appropriated in the 1921 Sheppard-Towner Maternity and Infancy Act. The Bureaus of Chemistry and Animal Industry in the Department of Agriculture were respectively charged with enforcing the 1906 Pure Food and Drugs Act and the 1906 Meat Inspection Act, a large public health responsibility. The Medical Division of the Office of Indian Affairs, St. Elizabeth's Hospital for the Insane, and Freedman's Hospital were all administered through the Interior Department. The War Department, in addition to providing medical services for its own personnel, administered the programs of the Veterans' Bureau.

Many other agencies had "an important but secondary interest in public health."[56] The Vital Statistics Division of the Bureau of the Census in the Department of Commerce was one example. In addition, there were "about twenty-five other federal agencies" that were "incidentally interested in public health," such as the Bureau of Immigration of the Labor Department. Tobey found that a total of five thousand medical, scientific, and nonprofessional personnel in the government were actually concerned with public health.[57] The amount allocated for the total public health effort in 1926, exclusive of meat inspections, was $11.6 million.[58] Tobey concluded:

> No one can study this situation without being convinced that it is, in general, an unsatisfactory one. The several services have been created, and they have had imposed upon them or have assumed their public health activities, in accordance with no carefully thought out plan. The result has been a diffusion of responsibility for the care of the public health, a failure in many cases to have an activity performed by that service which can perform it most efficiently and economically, and a duplication of activities, at least to the extent of a number of services doing work of precisely the same character.[59]

His proposal to remedy the situation was similar to that offered by the Committee of One Hundred nearly two decades before. "From a theoretical standpoint," Tobey said, "a strong argument might be made in favor of the establishment of a separate Department of Public Health."[60] He realized, however, that there was "strong opposition to the creation of new departments," and he therefore suggested that "the wiser course" would be to bring together "all federal services whose major activity lies in the field of public health" under the "common direction of an Assistant Secretary in one of the departments."[61] This was precisely the plan that former Surgeon General Rupert Blue had suggested to Senators Owen and Ransdell ten years earlier. Tobey, however, added a caveat designed to forestall opposition from nonorthodox medical groups like those that had defeated the efforts of the Committee of One Hundred. While it was certainly possible, said Tobey, for the "Surgeon General of the Public Health Service" to be "*ex officio* the assistant secretary for public health,*"* he stipulated that the person selected "need not be, and perhaps should not be, a physician,*"* though he should be "a person familiar with public health."[62]

At this point, the question should be raised about whether or not any changes in the existing structure of federal health agencies would have been as useful as Tobey and his associates proclaimed them to be. Certainly for citizens seeking information on health, it would have been easier to contact one agency than to find out which department handled a specific topic. On the other hand, the work of individual agencies had grown up because of their responsibilities to specific groups. Hence the Bureau of Indian Affairs, for example, dealt not only with the health needs of Indians but with other Indian concerns as well. The Children's Bureau was broadly concerned with the social welfare of children, which included their medical needs. And the Division of Vital Statistics of the Bureau of the Census was of importance in many areas besides public health.

In a 1927 study of the situation, Robert D. Leigh, a professor of government at Williams College, observed that in most reorganization schemes

> the task of reorganization has been looked upon as a single act of consolidating separate units. Their authors have seemed to regard bureaus and divisions as so many posts placed by statute in certain positions, to be pulled up and reset to satisfy a particular logic. In fact, they are much more like trees whose interlaced roots lie deep in the soil, whose transplanting is difficult if not disastrous, and whose growth is such that they need constant rather than intermittent attention. The rationale of the existing location of most services is found in day-to-day administrative operations and is usually hidden to paper reorganizers until their formulations meet the criticisms of the administrative agents affected.[63]

Leigh's perceptive comments reveal the way in which government agencies had been developed and are a key to understanding the opposition of many bureaucrats to consolidation schemes. For many purposes, coordination of personnel and resources between depart-

ments was more practical, but the prevailing emphasis on reorganization to achieve efficiency often caused advocates of consolidation to
ignore such observations. Tobey's proposals in *The National Government and Public Health,* which could have possibly resulted in the
consolidation of the Public Health Service, the Division of Vital Statistics, the Children's Bureau, the Bureaus of Chemistry and Animal
Industry, the Medical Division of the Office of Indian Affairs, St.
Elizabeth's Hospital for the Insane, and Freedman's Hospital into one
massive department of health, certainly contained one possible method
of organizing the health agencies of the federal government, a scheme
that was largely adopted in the late 1930s. Because of the disruption
to the interlaced roots of the bureaucratic tree, however, the proposals
were guaranteed to elicit opposition from the agencies that Tobey
proposed to transfer.

Leaders of the National Health Council had no reservations about
Tobey's proposals. They began active efforts to promote the plan in
the summer of 1925, before the book was published. Earlier that year
Tobey had editorialized in his column that Congress would "never give
to public health work the attention due it until there is in Washington
an avowed public health lobby which looks after the interests of san-
itarians, which are, of course, the interests of all the people, in the
same way that every other conceivable subject is promoted by duly
accredited agents in the Capitol."[64]

Tobey's suggestion was translated into an active group effort. In
July, Haley Fiske wrote to President Coolidge, attaching a summary
of Tobey's research. Fiske noted that Tobey's work would be finished
by November, at which time the committee hoped "to make some
concrete suggestions for your consideration."[65] The committee also
contacted Senator James W. Wadsworth, Jr., and found him favorable
to the idea.[66] Armed with the approval of the White House and at
least one senator, the committee sent "a representative of the American Medical Association to Washington to lobby" for a plan "by which
the various health activities would have been united under some lay
authority."[67] The attempt was defeated, according to Surgeon General
Hugh Cumming, "through the efforts of some of the leading health
authorities of the country."[68]

One of the major reasons for the rebuff of this effort was the
opposition of Public Health Service leaders to the reorganization plan.
Surgeon General Cumming had received a copy of the plan in the fall
of 1925 and was not at all pleased with the idea. Writing to Olin West,
secretary and general manager of the American Medical Association,
Cumming expressed disdain for "the so-called Institute for Government Research here (alias Willoughby and Tobey)" and "their mon-

strosity christened 'Tentative Plan for Coordination of Federal Health Activities.' "[69] The Surgeon General felt that Tobey had "done a very good piece of work in tracing out health activities in the Government but one which involved no particular mentality." In fact, he went on to say in another letter to C.-E.A. Winslow, then president of the American Public Health Association and member of the APHA committee supporting the proposal, "there were many of us who could have told him most of the things he found out. . . . He is not, I think, of broad vision."[70]

In response to the chilly reception given the proposal by leaders of the Service, the committee asked for Cumming's own ideas.[71] The Surgeon General seized this opportunity to set forth many of the changes the Service had desired since the 1912 act. He was aware that there was widespread support for the National Health Council's ideas and, unlike former Surgeon General Wyman, he chose to meld Service goals with the new proposals.[72] Moreover, Cumming had been pressed recently by a group of Service officers who reiterated their displeasure with the discrepancies in pay and perquisites between officers of the Public Health Service and those of the military.[73] Their complaint provided additional incentive to make a counterproposal that would advance the interests of the Service.

In consultation with other leaders of the Service, particularly with Assistant Surgeon General John Kerr, Cumming wrote a memorandum on the proposed reorganization. He summarized his plan:

> First, maintain the present organization of the Public Health Service; second, provide for admission into the regular corps of scientific men other than those of the medical profession similar to the corps of the Foreign Service of our Government; third, enact legislation authorizing the head of the Public Health Service to detail personnel for public health duties in other Departments of the Government, thus solving the difficulty with reference to bureaus only partly devoted to medical subjects such as the Children's Bureau; fourth, provide for the transfer of the Division of Vital Statistics to the Public Health Service.[74]

Tobey and his associates agreed to the changes proposed by Cumming. These suggestions, which also included making the Hygienic Laboratory Advisory Board a National Advisory Health Council, were incorporated into the final draft of *The National Government and Public Health* and were published as part of Tobey's recommendations.[75] In January 1926 members of the American Public Health Association committee visited President Coolidge to discuss the proposals.[76] Coolidge suggested that a bill be prepared embodying the recommendations. Having received the president's blessing, Tobey began work with a Public Health Service representative and a lawyer from the House of Representatives legislative drafting service. They "incorporated all the proposals into a patchwork quilt of a bill."[77] On March 8, 1926, New York congressman James S. Parker introduced the bill, H.R. 10125, into the House of Representatives.[78] Parker, chairman of the House Committee on Interstate and Foreign Commerce, to which the bill would be referred, had sponsored the legislation at the request of the Service. Parker had no personal interest in the bill, and indeed, he does not appear to have worked for its passage to any extent.

The proposals of the National Health Council were contained in section one of the bill. It authorized the president to transfer by executive order of the Public Health Service any other executive agency engaged in health work, except those of the military. Section two was a companion measure that reflected the Service's approach to coordination of health agencies. Instead of consolidation, this provision allowed the president to detail officers or employees of the Service to other executive agencies "in order to supervise or cooperate in" work pertaining to public health. The Surgeon General could also detail officers if he was so requested by the agency to which the officers were to be sent.

Sections five and seven dealt with the personnel problems of the Service. Section five stated that sanitary engineers, dental officers, and scientists would become commissioned officers, "selected for general service and subject to changes of station." A Service memorandum on this provision of the bill underscored the need for commissioning sanitary engineers, noting their important contributions to the control of epidemics after major disasters such as floods.[79] This section also provided that the Surgeon General be raised to the equivalent rank of the Surgeon General of the Army for purposes of pay and allowances. All members of the Commissioned Officers Corps, moreover, were to be promoted at a rate comparable to their counterparts in the Medical Corps of the Army, and the existing limitation on the number of Assistant Surgeons General and Senior Surgeons in the Service was to be repealed. Assistant Surgeons General engaged in field service were to be designated Medical Directors.

A nurse corps was authorized to be created by section seven. The Service already employed 354 nurses whose duties were "comparable to those of the Army and Navy."[80] These nurses, however, lacked the benefits of those in the military because they were Civil Service employees, while military nurses had their own nurse corps. This situation naturally led many Public Health Service nurses to seek transfer to the Army or Navy.

Sections three and eight of the Parker bill addressed the Hygienic Laboratory. The increasing complexity of scientific research was recognized in section 3(a), which allowed medical and scientific personnel to be detailed to universities and research institutes "for special studies of scientific problems relating to public health and for the dissemination of information relating to public health." If enacted, this provision would give official sanction to the cancer research program underway at Harvard. A reciprocal arrangement would allow research personnel at nongovernmental laboratories to use the Hygienic Laboratory when necessary in research projects. "Research," the Service memorandum on this provision noted, "is becoming more difficult . . . and requires greater coordination for its successful performance, both on the part of official and unofficial agencies."[81] The proposed exchange program would allow the government to "utilize scientific equipment and facilities which, were they provided by the government, would cost many thousands of dollars."[82] This section also extended the facilities of the Hygienic Laboratory to state and local health authorities, a practice that had been in effect to a limited degree for years but without official sanction.

Section 3(b) authorized the secretary of the Treasury to establish additional divisions in the Hygienic Laboratory as he deemed "necessary to provide agencies for the solution of public health problems." William H. Welch, longtime member of the Hygienic Laboratory Advisory Board, commenting later at hearings on the bill, expressed surprise that anyone should question the need for this sort of flexibility. He observed that "as knowledge grows, various branches of scientific study are developed."[83] Section eight provided that the Advisory Board of the Hygienic Laboratory be renamed the National Advisory Health Council, authorized the Surgeon General to increase the board's membership by five members, and stated that the board could "advise the Surgeon General of the Public Health Service in respect of public health activities."

The remaining sections of the Parker bill were assigned to correct administrative difficulties within the Service. Section six updated an archaic rule that hindered the Service from acting quickly in an emergency. Under Treasury Department regulations, the secretary of the Treasury had to approve in writing the appointment of any employee before he or she began work. During an outbreak of plague in New Orleans, this had meant that "it was necessary to telegraph more than one hundred names to Washington" of local people needed to assist in supressing the outbreak and waiting for their names to be "telegraphed again to the field before the employees could be placed on duty."[84] As a corrective measure, the Parker bill allowed the Treasury secretary to approve the names retroactively to the date on which they began employment. Section 4(a) provided that estimates should be submitted on the cost of consolidating the various offices and laboratories of the Service into a central facility. These offices were at that time scattered throughout the District of Columbia. Section 4(b) defined for administrative purposes the Hygienic Laboratory as a field station of the Service, even though it was located in Washington.

The Parker bill was wide ranging in its provisions, the most complete reorganization proposal since the 1902 act. Anticipating the questions that the bill would raise from H. M. Lord, the director of the Budget who was not perceived as friendly to Service interests but whose approval was necessary for any bill to receive serious consideration, Surgeon General Cumming initialled two memoranda prepared by Assistant Surgeon General John Kerr explaining what additional costs would be incurred and how many personnel would be affected.[85] The memorandum on costs stated that a net increase of $9,500 in salaries would be required. The commissioning of dentists, sanitary engineers, and scientists would cost $22,000, but the creation of a nurse corps would effect a decrease of $13,000. This decrease would occur because the initial salaries of commissioned nurses would be lower than under Civil Service regulations. To the nurses advocating commissioned status, however, lower initial salaries were offset by the benefits inherent in a commission: regular raises in pay, job security, and retirement benefits not available to civil servants. An additional $500 would be required for compensation of the new members of the National Advisory Health Council. All other provisions of the bill entailed no additional cost. The small increase of $9,500, the memorandum maintained, "would be offset many times by the intangible savings and increase of efficiency that would result." The memorandum on personnel noted that the total number of people affected would be "about 246, all of whom" already held positions within the Service.

The Parker bill was referred to the House Committeee on Interstate and Foreign Commerce, where it languished for lack of approval from the Budget Bureau. In May 1926 Tobey visited John Kerr to inquire about General Lord's objections.[86] Tobey was under the impression that Lord objected only to the personnel changes contained in the bill. Kerr, who recently had conferred with Lord, reported that the Budget director was "broadly in favor of coordination," but objected not only to the "extension of commissions to other than physicians" but also to increasing the pay of commissioned officers. The bill, therefore, remained in committee throughtout the summer and fall. Service leaders secured the approval of Treasury Secretary Andrew Mellon, but they could not budge Lord.[87]

In his column in the September 1926 issue of the *American Journal of Public Health* Tobey commented dryly on the situation: "This measure failed to receive the sanction of the czar of the Budget, one General H. M. Lord. Although Mr. Lord approved numerous bills carrying many times the expense that this bill did, he balked at a paltry sum of about $10,000 a year for public health, on the alleged grounds that this was 'contrary to the President's financial policy,' whatever that means. Many sanitarians are convinced that his failure to approve this bill is, to say the least, disingenuous."[88] Surgeon General Cumming put the matter more bluntly. In a letter to one of his Service colleagues in New Orleans, Cumming stated: "General Lord's statement . . . about it being impossible to increase [the number of] commissions, etc. in any branch of the Service was not borne out by the passage of the Coast Guard or Navy personnel bills and I am agraid that his real objection is because of his attitude toward the medical profession."[89]

By the end of the year, the tension between Service officials and the Bureau of the Budget threatened to become a public battle. Lord telephoned Cumming in December "to ask if he knew of any controversy" between them, because "a *New York Times* reporter" was circulating such a rumor.[90] Perhaps wondering if his frank statements to friends had not remained confidential, Cumming told Lord "he was unable to recall any circumstances that would give this impression." John Kerr, who recorded this conversation in a memorandum, noted that General Lord remained "entirely cordial" and that the rumor was quelled.

Although in 1926 the future did not look bright for the Parker bill, the mere existnece of such a bill marked the first time the Service had joined forces with public health leaders to accomplish both internal reforms and a greater overall centralization of federal health work. It should be noted that this alliance was more expedient than committed. The members of the national health movement could not afford the open opposition of the Public Health Service, and the Service had repeatedly failed to accomplish by itself desired internal reorganization. This alliance reflected a recognition by the national health movement that their ends would have to be reached through the vehicle of the existing Public Health Service. Thus was the fifty-year-old campaign for a centralized public health agency melded with the most powerful bureaucracy among those dealing with health matters.

The provisions of the Parker bill affecting the Hygienic Laboratory were considered an integral part of the new proposal, but the Laboratory itself was still viewed as the research arm of a broader effort that included preventive measures, public education, and some health care delivery. Because of this broad orientation of the Service and the national health movement, there was no major effort to increase significantly the size and scope of activity in the Hygienic Laboratory other than the specific reforms included in the bill. Paralleling the activities of the Service and the national health movement, however, was another movement in the scientific community that came to focus its efforts solely on the size and direction of the Hygienic Laboratory. This movement produced a companion bill to the Parker bill that sought to transform the Hygienic Laboratory into a National Institute of Health. Before proceeding further, therefore, consideration must be given to the development of this second proposal and the rise of the scientific research community as a major force in federal health policy.

PART TWO

Origins in World War I Scientific Research

FOUR

Dr. Herty Proposes an Institute
for Drug Research

> One of the most surprising outcomes of the war has been
> the sudden and I believe permanent enthronement of science in the
> activities of humanity.
> —*Glenn W. Herrick, 1920*

our months after the Parker bill was introduced, a second
bill, which proposed an enormous expansion of medical research in the Public Health Service, was laid before the
Congress. Sponsored by Louisiana senator Joseph Eugene
Ransdell, this bill sought the creation of a National Institute of Health
in which the "fundamental problems" of the diseases of man would be
studied. It included an initial appropriation of $15 million for a five-
year period to construct buildings and support research.

The Ransdell bill, with its provision for vastly augmented expenditures for medical research by the federal government, grew out of
the proposal for a private-sector research institute made by a group
of scientists who believed that basic scientific research was the key
to medical advances in the twentieth century. Their conviction was
rooted in the so-called pure-science ideal of the nineteenth century.
This doctrine rejected usefulness as a rationale for scientific activities,
requiring instead that "knowledge should be evaluated according to
its significance for existing theory and in no other terms" and that
"scientists should be evaluated solely on the basis of their contributions
to knowledge."[1]

Taking the German university system that emphasized laboratory
research as their model, these scientists pressed with limited success
for the establishment of pure or basic science in American universities.
Their efforts also to install the new ideal in the scientific bureaus of
the federal government were rebuffed, at least in the congressionally
mandated missions assigned to scientific bureaus. The United States
government had supported a number of scientific activities in the
nineteenth century, including the Lewis and Clark expedition, a Coast

Survey, and a Geological survey. These activities, however, were predicated on obtaining practical results — information on new regions, aids for maritime commerce, and the discovery of mineral wealth that could be economically exploited. Scientists involved in these undertakings were increasingly aware that theoretical or pure science advances were needed in order to accomplish some of their goals. Mapping projects, for instance, often required celestial observations, which in turn posed questions about astronomy.[2] Congress, as A. Hunter Dupree has pointed out, understood that the complexities of pure science were important though not easily understood by nonscientists. Nonetheless, as officers of the government, congressmen were accountable for expenditures of public funds. This yoke of responsibility severely limited any expansion of federal support into wholly theoretical areas.[3]

By the Progressive Era, the scientific community had come to the conclusion that basic science was properly housed in academia and that government scientific activities would be limited to utilitarian purposes for the specific good of society. For two decades this system worked fairly well. Individuals, professional associations, and voluntary associations contributed to the establishment of research funds in universities.[4] The burgeoning growth of the scientific community that occurred in the twentieth century was in its infancy during the Progressive Era. Hence demands for laboratory space, equipment, and assistance could be met within this existing structure.

To finance more ambitious projects, scientists turned to philanthropists and foundations. Andrew Carnegie endowed the Carnegie Institution of Washington in 1902 for research in the physical sciences. The previous year, medical research advanced by a quantum leap with the establishment of the Rockefeller Institute for Medical Research in New York. Opened in 1906, the Rockefeller Institute was extremely important to medical research for two reasons. It created a model in the minds of scientists and the public alike that private philanthropy was the appropriate source for research funds. It also adopted the ideal of pure laboratory research. The institute's staff members were relieved of any obligation to teach or engage in routine duties; they were afforded the best equipment and technical support available; and their sole goal was to be the advancement of knowledge.[5]

Other privately endowed research institutes followed the example of the Rockefeller, although no other equaled its scale. Most of these other institutes were devoted to work on a particular disease or group of related maladies. In 1902 Harold F. McCormick established the John Rockefeller McCormick Memorial Institute for Infectious Diseases in Chicago. McCormick, heir to the agricultural machinery fortune, was motivated in part by the death of his eldest son as a result of scarlet fever, an incurable disease at that time.[6] Such personal tragedies also played a part in other philanthropic grants, as did a philosophy of stewardship of the great fortunes accumulated in this period. Thus the Hooper Institute for Medical Research was established in San Francisco; the Phipps Institute for the study, treatment, and prevention of tuberculosis was opened in Philadelphia; the Cushing Institute in Cleveland; Trudeau's tuberculosis laboratory at Sarnac; and the Otho S. A. Sprague Institute for Infectious Diseases in Chicago.

The word *institute*, however, was used loosely. Many institutes were begun as separate entities only to become a part of a university, as the Phipps Institute did, joining the University of Pennsylvania in 1910, only seven years after it was established. The cost of construction of new facilities and the necessity of providing a large endowment fostered the growth of smaller scale "institutes" that retained some degree of autonomy but were still a part of their respective universities.

On the eve of World War I the relationship among science, the private sector, and the government was in a state of equilibrium, the private sector supporting basic research as well as applied work and the federal government devoting its revenues to practical scientific work. The Great War was a watershed that marked the beginnings of destabilizing this equilibrium. Problems generated by the war revealed the indispensability of science, both pure and applied, to national defense and the general welfare. By the war's end, public appreciation for science had increased dramatically. In 1920, for instance, Glenn W. Herrick of Cornell University told his institution's new initiates of Sigma Xi, an honorary scientific research society, that "one of the most surprising outcomes of the war has been the sudden and I believe permanent enthronement of science in the activities of humanity."[7]

Before World War I the United States had for years relied on German pharmaceuticals, dyestuffs, munitions, and other products of German organic chemical research. The outbreak of war in 1914 interrupted international trade and led to a reassessment of the need for systematic support in America for research and development. In industry, for example, some smaller firms followed the precedent of such large firms as American Telephone and Telegraph Company and General Electric Company in establishing in-house research laboratories.[8] The National Academy of Sciences likewise responded to the situation by creating a National Research Council at the urging of George Ellery Hale, director of the Mt. Wilson Observatory, member of the National Academy of Sciences, and tireless promoter of science.[9] The council's mission was to bring together and mobilize academic, governmental, and industrial scientists for national defense. It had quickly become clear, Hale wrote after the war, "that many of the problems of war lie in the domain of the physicist, the chemist, the meteorologist, no less than in that of the military expert."[10]

Although scientists from many disciplines contributed to the war effort, World War I was often regarded as "a chemist's war," and it was out of the experience of chemists in the war that proposals developed leading to the Ransdell bill for a National Institute of Health. One writer, reflecting in 1920 on the wartime contributions of chemists, noted that at the "beginning of the war in 1914, there were no indications that the chemist would be of any more value than in previous wars."[11] On April 22, 1915, however, the Germans bombarded Allied lines at Ypres with canisters of chlorine gas, a weapon against which conventional protective devices were useless. Gas warfare suddenly demanded the expertise of the chemist to develop counter gasses, gas masks and, in cooperation with physiologists and pharmacologists, treatment for the victims of gas attacks.

In the United States, which in 1915 remained neutral, a number of leaders of the scientific community promoted precautionary measures that would prepare the military for gas warfare in case the country became involved in the hostilities. The first task undertaken was a census of American chemists. This was a cooperative effort in 1916 by the newly formed National Research Council and the American Chemical Society (ACS). Because 14,500 out of 17,000 chemists in the United States belonged to the ACS, the society was able to provide information about the fields of expertise of most American chemists that could be utilized by the government as need arose.[12] Directing this census for the ACS was Charles Holmes Herty, who in 1916 was serving his second term as president of the society.

In 1917, when the census of chemists was complete, Herty became the first full-time editor of the society's *Journal of Industrial and Engineering Chemistry*. From this position he was able to publicize the work of chemists in the war, and after the formation of the Chemical Warfare Service in July 1918, he ran a series of articles in the *Journal* entitled "Contributions from the Chemical Warfare Service."[13] Herty and other chemists were especially impressed with the problem-solving approach taken by this agency.[14] Instead of relying on the possible results of individuals working in isolation, the Service organized research teams and assigned each a particular aspect of the larger problem to be solved. Many of these teams were located at "branch laboratories" in cooperating institutions; others were concentrated in a major research center established at the American University Experiment Station in Washington, D.C. Daniel P. Jones described the cooperative process in this way:

A sample of the new compound was prepared by one team, then its physical and chemical properties were studied by another team to determine its stability in shell casings, its volatility, etc. Meanwhile, a unit of the pharmacological section examined its biological effects. A meeting was then arranged between the chemists, physiologists, and pharmacologists involved, to decide if the compound was suitable for use in combat. If so, the task of developing a small-scale manufacturing process was given to another section, and at the same time a sample of the compound was examined by the defense section to ensure that American gas masks could be modified to give adequate protection against this compound. If all investigations to this point gave satisfactory results, the project was submitted to the Development Division or directly to the Gas Manufacturing Division of the Chemical Warfare Service. Often the chemists who were most familiar with the new agent were transferred to these divisions with the project.[15]

The rapidity and efficiency with which tasks could be accomplished in such a framework led many chemists and other scientists to press for greater coordination of research in peacetime. At the war's end many of them wrote and lectured about the opportunities at hand and the benefits to be gained from increasing cooperative research. Burton E. Livingston of the Johns Hopkins University argued, for example, that scientists must abandon "the extremely individualistic methods of the Middle Ages," and adopt a cooperative spirit, which he defined as "the union of a number of minds in planning the attack on a problem, in working out the different parts, and in bringing the several component results together into a well-considered presentation that might really mark a tangible advance in scientific knowledge."[16]

Proponents of the cooperative ideal were aware of the hurdles presented by the geographical distance between scientists who might potentially collaborate, by the need for adequate funding to make cooperative ventures possible, and by the problem of determining the merits of proposals suggested. Livingston outlined a model in which a central committee, under the auspices of the National Research Council, would review proposals and disperse funds, but he did not identify a source for the funds. Many scientists, especially George Ellery Hale, encouraged an increase in donations from industry and private philanthropy for this purpose.[17]

Among the scientists who promoted cooperative research was Charles Holmes Herty. His involvement with the Chemical Warfare Service convinced him that cooperative, project-oriented research offered great promise for the development of new pharmaceutical agents. The medical problems of the war and the influenza pandemic of 1918 pointed up the fact that little progress had been made in chemotherapy since Paul Ehrlich's 1910 discovery of salvarsan as a specific for syphilis. Ehrlich, who had predicted in 1913 that many more "magic bullets" would be found, had focused his efforts on infectious diseases. Herty and his associates in chemistry and pharmacology sought to broaden the definition of chemotherapy to include "all types of substances used in therapeutics."[18]

In the summer of 1918 Herty and University of Texas organic chemist J. R. Bailey discussed the potential application of cooperative research to medicine as they made their way home from a baseball game in New York City.[19] "Perched upon an iron railing amidst the upper Broadway crowds," Herty and Bailey analyzed the problem. They recognized the fact that other applications of the newly developing American synthetic organic chemical industry, explosives and dyestuffs, were economically profitable to those who invested in research and development on them. Pharmaceutical firms, however, rarely undertook the study of chemical compounds for their potential as new medicinals. What Herty believed was possible to remedy this situation was the establishment of an institute, "in which laboratory tests of all kinds would be made and to which, through the establishment of fellowships, manufacturing organizations could send well-trained young men for working out specific problems. Cooperation could be established between this institution and the organic laboratories of our universities, as well as with the hospitals of the country."[20]

In August Herty wrote to some of the most distinguished members of the medical research community about his idea. He discussed the idea with P. A. Levine and Simon Flexner of the Rockefeller Institute, and found them "enthusiastic over the proposition."[21] He also wrote to John J. Abel, the noted pharmacologist at the Johns Hopkins University. Abel also supported the idea but emphasized that cooperation between chemists and pharmacologists should be stressed.[22]

Herty used his position as editor of the *Journal of Industrial and Engineering Chemistry* as a platform for this idea. He published an unsigned editorial in the September 1918 issue suggesting the establishment of a privately endowed facility for drug research similar to the Mellon Institute for Industrial Research. To counter suggestions that such work could best be carried on in universities, drug firms, or government laboratories, Herty stated:

> In university circles there is often lacking that spirit of cooperation between the several classes of research workers which would insure a thorough

examination of these new products of the organic chemical laboratory, or, if the spirit be willing, the means for conducting the tests are too limited, especially now when university finances are so severely contracted. In a few manufacturing establishments provision is made for animal experimentation, but these facilities are entirely inadequate and not available to all organic chemists. In government laboratories some provision is made for this work, but restrictions are enforced by inadequate appropriations. And still people suffer.[23]

When Herty published this editorial, he was at the pinnacle of a distinguished career in applied chemistry. He was born December 4, 1867, in Milledgeville, Georgia, the same year that Joseph Lister introduced antiseptic surgery to the world.[24] He was the older of the two children of Louisa Turno Holmes and Bernard Ritchie Herty. His father, who had been a captain in the Confederate army, was a druggist; both parents died before Herty was nine years old. He and his sister were reared by an aunt. He obtained his undergraduate education at the University of Georgia, taking his bachelor's degree in 1886. He then went to Baltimore, Maryland, intending to spend a year strengthening his knowledge of chemistry at the Johns Hopkins University. The noted chemist Ira Remsen convinced the brash young man that he needed more rigorous training, and Herty remained to take his Ph.D. with Remsen in 1890.

In 1891 Herty took a position in the chemistry department at the University of Georgia. In addition to teaching, the avid sports fan brought Glenn "Pop" Warner and the game of football to the university. Herty remained at the University of Georgia for eight years, during which time he married Sophie Schaller, who came from a prominent Athens family. In 1899 he took leave to study at the Universities of Zurich and Berlin, institutions notable for work in applied chemistry, pharmacy, and forestry. In Zurich Herty worked with the future Nobel laureate in chemistry, Alfred Werner, and in Berlin with the synthetic dye chemist Otto N. Witt. Out of this period of study came the first of Herty's achievements in applied chemistry. When Witt characterized the American method of carving a box in pine trees to harvest the gum as "butchery of the pines," Herty resolved to investigate the charge.[25] His research led to the development of the cup and gutter method of turpentining; his cooperation with the Chattanooga Pottery Company in producing "Herty cups" made him financially independent. The Herty cup "resulted in savings to the naval stores industry, reducing the evaporation of turpentine and the coloration of the resin, diminished forest fires, and raised the quality of the lumber subsequently harvested."[26]

From 1905 to 1916 Herty served as professor of chemistry and dean of the School of Applied Science at the University of North Carolina. It was during his tenure in North Carolina that he served two terms as president of the American Chemical Society, in 1915 and 1916. Upon assuming the editorship of the *Journal* in 1917, Herty turned his considerable talent as a speaker and writer to the advancement of chemistry and the chemical industry in America and to the broader goal of cooperation in science.[27] His editorial calling for a cooperative institute for drug research was one part of this effort.

Response to the editorial, which Herty had solicited from readers, was quickly forthcoming. H.A.B. Dunning, a chemist and partner in the Baltimore drug firm of Hynson, Westcott and Dunning, wrote that the proposed cooperation between academic and commercial pharmacologists might be hard to get. He noted that university pharmacologists considered it "non-ethical to do work for industrial concerns," an attitude that had its roots in the policy of the American Society of Pharmacology and Therapeutics to exclude from membership permanent employees of drug firms.[28] This policy, of which John J. Abel was a leading exponent, was a response to the sometimes shameless exploitation of "experts" by commercial firms. As one authority put it: "The lack of cooperation which has existed between men in university chairs and manufacturing concerns has been due to many factors. The university man had to feel absolutely certain that his name and university connection would not be used in any way for advertising purposes . . . . [M]any of our best drug firms have been in the habit of making unwarranted statements in their advertising which were not borne out by the facts."[29] Any institute created for research on drugs would have to find a workable solution to this problem.

A different response came from the *Philadelphia Public Ledger*. The paper was enthusiastic about Herty's proposal, but suggested in an editorial on the subject that "this proposed laboratory" be "made a part of the existing National Bureau of Standards which already" covered "certain phases of chemistry in its physical determinations."[30] The *Ledger* acknowledged, however, that the chemists would "probably want their own laboratory," and that the need for one was unquestioned.

Herty planned to publish these and other responses in the November issue of the *Journal*, but he was convinced by "a number of prominent men who" had "become very much interested in the subject" first to devote a meeting of the New York section of the American Chemical Society to his proposal and print those addresses in the *Journal*.[31] Herty was chairman of the New York section, so the decision to make the institute the topic of the November meeting was swiftly reached.

Invitations were extended to prominent chemists and pharmacologists, and the symposium took place on November 8. In addition to endorsing the establishment of the institute, the speakers addressed the critical problems of its organization and mission. Which fundamental research problems were appropriate to be studied? What relationship should the institute develop with manufacturing firms? How should power be shared among the different professional groups involved? How should the institute be financed to maintain integrity and independence?

Pharmacologist John J. Abel, who sent a letter because he was unable to attend, chose to designate the proposed institute "A National Institute for Drug Research."[32] He stressed the need to perform pharmacological research, such as the isolation of hormones and the synthesizing of drugs already known. P. A. Levine, a biochemist at the Rockefeller Institute for Medical Research, envisioned "An Institute for Chemotherapy." He suggested a more broadly conceived facility with two aims: theoretical work in medicinal chemistry by a permanent staff from a variety of disciplines and applied work for short periods of time by manufacturing firms needing to solve particular problems. A. S. Loevenhart, a pharmacologist engaged in chemical warfare work at the American University Experiment Station, proposed "An Institute for Research in Synthetic Organic Chemistry." Stressing the productivity stimulated by cooperation between chemists and pharmacologists during World War I, Loevenhart envisioned a complex facility that would serve as a chemical resource center, regulatory agency, and research laboratory. He proposed that the institute maintain "the largest possible collection of organic chemicals which would be furnished to any university or industrial concern at cost, synthesize for American chemists any substances required for their work, obtain and administer patents claimed by organic chemists, and perform final therapeutic tests on any new drugs in an adjoining hospital devoted to experimental therapy."[33]

Two representatives of manufacturing firms also spoke about an institute. Frank R. Eldred of Eli Lilly and Company urged that basic research be the focus of a "Therapo-chemical" institute so that "the actual mechanism" of drug action in the body could be elucidated and then integrated with pharmacology in an informed manner, "rather than along the more superficial lines usually thought of in connection with pharmacological work."[34] He stressed that the greatest need was not for more drugs but for better and fewer drugs. Both he and D. W. Jayne of the Barret Company emphasized the need for cooperation between academic scientists and industrial producers of drugs, especially in regard to the question of patent rights to new drugs. Eldred said: "The drug manufacturer must receive the full measure of protection accorded to other manufacturers. He must not be discriminated against in the matter of patent protection as has been advocated in certain quarters. No other factor could be more potent in preventing progress in this branch of industry than the elimination of product claims from chemical patents."[35]

All speakers agreed that the institute should be under private auspices, but most supported the concept of cooperation with government agencies. C. L. Alsberg, chief of the Bureau of Chemistry in the Department of Agriculture, predicted that "the work of his bureau would dovetail into the work of the proposed institute."[36] The Bureau of Chemistry investigated possible violation by patent medicine manufacturers under the Pure Food and Drugs Act and analyzed nonbiologic medicinals as well. Research by a private institute could have assisted this government effort by identifying and testing potentially useful drugs.

Estimates of the endowment needed to establish the institute varied. Loevenhart projected "at least $1,000,000, but preferably not less than $5,000,000."[37] Abel, writing to Herty shortly after the meeting, also believed it would require a "number of millions." What was needed, said Abel, was some "old millionaire who is about to join his ancestors and wishes to put his millions to the best possible use."[38] Abel also pointed out the danger of beginning with too little money. "The only fear in my mind," his letter continued, "is that we shall not raise enough money to have anything more than a testing place for firms."

After hearing the addresses at its November meeting, the New York section endorsed Herty's idea and passed a resolution urging that "such an institute should be under the general guidance of the American Chemical Society."[39] This resolution was sent to the Advisory Committee of the society. In response, the Advisory Committee authorized president William Nichols "to appoint a committee to report to the Advisory Committee a statement of endowment needed for salaries, buildings, equipment and operating expenses, and an outline of policies for such an institute."[40] Herty was named chairman of the committee and was requested to suggest names for the other committee members. Of the people he suggested, all of whom were approved, three had presented addresses at the November symposium: John J. Abel, Frank R. Eldred, and P. A. Levine.[41] Other members were Raymond F. Bacon, director of the Mellon Institute for Industrial Research; Reid Hunt, pharmacologist at Harvard Medical School; Treat B. Johnson, Yale University chemist; F. O. Taylor, chief chemist for Parke, Davis and Company; and, after April 1920,

Julius Stieglitz, chairman of the department of chemistry at the University of Chicago.[42]

Even before the committee was appointed, however, rivalries erupted over control of the proposed institute. Research into medicinal drugs overlapped the disciplines of chemistry, pharmacy, and medicine, and representatives of each promoted the leadership merits of his own discipline. Edward Kremers, director of the pharmaceutical program at the University of Wisconsin, wrote to Frank Eldred: "Why should American pharmaceutical manufacturers support an institution fostered by the Am. Chem. Society when pharmaceutical institutions are in the greatest need of all the financial support in sight. I trust that our pharmaceutical manufacturers will prove true to their own calling first . . . . Is the American Pharmaceutical Association going to take a back seat another time and allow the A.C.S. to do its work?"[43]

Eldred was annoyed that the pharmacists believed they "ought to have something to do with a movement which they have been thinking about for twenty years, but have failed to initiate." It was, he went on in a letter to Herty, "rather amusing to see how aggrieved they are to find that someone has acted while they were thinking about the matter."[44] Eldred, obviously no admirer of the American Pharmaceutical Association, proposed that "an effort be made to strengthen the Division of Pharmaceutical Chemistry of the A.C.S. and bring it to the point where it will be fully representative of scientific pharmacy."

The opposition of pharmacists to American Chemical Society control of the proposed institute was mere aggravation compared with the perceived threat posed by the American Medical Association (AMA). In the April 1919 issue of the *Chicago Chemical Bulletin*, an editorial writer asserted that the AMA should be consulted and have a prominent part in the proposed institution's organization and management.[45] John M. Francis of Parke, Davis and Company expressed the dire concern of the pharmaceutical manufacturers over possible AMA control. He denounced the directors of the association to Herty, claiming that

> the ultimate aim of this small body of governing men in this association looks to, or at least is desirous of, dominating everything that pertains to medicine, surgery, pharmacy and the allied branches. They want to dominate not only in private life but are even ambitious enough to look forward to domination in Congressional and state legislation and in the Army and Navy and the various government institutions. It is very natural, therefore, for me to say to you frankly that the pharmaceutical manufacturers of this country and many others as well, look with distrust and anxiety upon any arrangement which would allow official appointees of the A.M.A. to play

too prominent a part in the organization and government of this proposed institute.[46]

The reason for such strongly worded opposition to AMA involvement had to do with changes in the association's goals stemming from its 1901 reorganization. At that time its power base shifted from public health leaders and medical school professors to general practitioners. Coupled with the association's success in raising the profession's standards and economic status, this shift made the AMA the "chief spokesman for private medicine."[47] The association had recently defeated an attempt to enact compulsory health insurance in the United States, and it was noted for its desire to dominate all activities related to medicine. Its Council on Pharmacy and Chemistry, which had been established in 1905 to analyze the ingredients in proprietary products, would certainly be interested in any institute on drug research.[48]

The objections of physicians and pharmacologists to control of any institute by the American Chemical Society was not merely the result of interdisciplinary rivalry, however. John Parascandola has pointed out that the AMA's Council of Pharmacy and Chemistry was "wary of the pharmaceutical and chemical industries," and that the ACS was "closely identified with the chemical industry" at this time. Objections of pharmacists grew out of concern that many scientists, especially chemists, "failed to acknowledge pharmacy as a branch of science."[49]

As the committee deliberated, Herty's skills as a diplomat were tested in smoothing ruffled feathers in these disputes. He quickly found out who had written the editorial that dismayed Francis and was assured by "a prominent member" of the Chicago section of the AMA that committee members should "pay no official attention to it."[50] The task of guiding the committee to consensus on an organizational hierarchy for the institute presented similar problems. At the first committee meeting on February 22, 1919, there was apparently a wide-ranging discussion of this topic, because a flurry of correspondence between Herty and committee members followed. Frank Eldred complained that neither P. A. Levine nor John J. Abel "seemed to have the conception of complete cooperation between members of the staff which is the fundamental idea of our project."[51] Abel had proposed that a physical chemist work under the direction of a pharmacologist, although he wondered whether an eminent physical chemist could be expected to devote himself to biological problems. Eldred also attacked Levine's conception of an institute organized along the lines of the Rockefeller Institute. "I think," Eldred opined, "that a little investigation of the work of the [Rockefeller] institution will show that there is a surprising lack of cooperation between the various departments of the institute."[52] Plainly the ideal of selfless cooperation in the service of scientific research was not easily reconciled with the desire for status among individual scientists.

Overshadowing all other questions relating to the institute, however, was the problem of raising money to endow it. Committee members differed over the scale on which the institute should be started and the methods used to acquire funds, although all agreed that the source of funds should be a wealthy individual. Eldred believed that "an endowment of $2,000,000 or even $1,000,000 would be sufficient for the establishment of the institution, if some provision existed by which this endowment might be increased when the work of the institute grew to such proportions as to require it."[53] He believed in starting small, perhaps leasing a building in which to begin work. Herty disagreed. "If the work is really important work," he wrote Eldred, "it should be done by the best men in the country . . . . Now of course it would be a decided waste of the energies of these men if they had to work without sufficient assistance, and so the necessity of the larger staff naturally follows."[54]

The method by which to secure the endowment was also the subject of some debate. P. A. Levine, adopting a strategy that had been employed in founding the Rockefeller Institute, proposed "quietly seeking the man and laying the matter before him, and talking about the matter after the endowment had been secured."[55] Herty, in contrast, believed that there should be an active program of public education on the need for the institute. He felt that "sentiment must be developed among chemists, and the general public must become sympathetic, and become convinced of the benefits to be received, and when they do become convinced I am sure that somewhere in this general public we shall find a man or men who will give us the money."[56] He added that he did not "expect this to be an easy task, or one which" would be "quickly finished."

In March 1919 the committee drafted a tentative outline for the proposed institute. Its mission was to be "the study of the fundamental problems connected with the living body (whose every change is fundamentally a chemical change)."[57] Such an orientation placed the committee in the tradition of Jacques Loeb and his followers, who promoted a mechanistic view of life.[58] To accomplish its mission the institute was to be organized into three major divisions: chemistry, pharmacology, and experimental biology. Seven subdivisions within these major areas each would be headed by a chief whose salary was set at $12,000. There would also be a director, administrative staff, seven "associates" for the divisions, twenty-one assistant scientists, and ninety-five technicians and "helpers." The permanent staff would be

devoted to pure research. Drug manufacturers were to be offered the
facilities for solution of their particular problems; the drug firms were
expected to finance this work through the creation of industrial fellowships similar to those at the Mellon Institute. The annual operating
costs were projected at $420,000, which represented the interest at
5 percent on $8.4 million. After including an additional $2 million for
the cost of buildings and grounds, the committee recommended seeking an endowment of $10.4 million. Control of the institute was to be
"vested in two distinct bodies, the one financial and the other scientific." Members of the financial board were to be "the ablest financiers
in the country." The scientific board was to consist of "seven men
preeminent in the subjects represented in the seven divisions of the
scientific staff, and one member elected annually by the Advisory
Committee of the American Chemical Society."[59]

The deliberations of the committee had led to a more broadly conceived institute than Herty had envisioned in the 1918 editorial. The
basic research proposed was nothing less than articulation of the chemical mechanisms of the human body. Excited about such a challenge,
John M. Francis wrote to Herty that this kind of basic research had
"received little attention at the hands of scientists either in America
or Europe" but would "constitute the real basis for all advance along
the lines of therapeutic development." He suggested broadening the
title of the institute to one for "Physiologic Chemistry," by which he
meant "the chemistry involved in the reactions which take place between the protoplasm of the animal body when brought into contact
with the thousand and one substances which have medicinal or therapeutic effect." Francis anticipated the magnitude of the problems to
be faced in unraveling the chemical functions of the body. "As one
begins to think it over," he mused, "the field becomes enormous,
involving all the various body secretions and their constitution and the
chemical changes which they undergo in different portions of the body."
Almost uncannily foreshadowing the development of the National Institutes of Health after World War II, Francis observed: "Of course
if you are going to combine physiologic chemistry with 'Pharmaceutical
Chemistry,' pharmacological, bacteriological and clinical testing, you
have in mind a still greater institution; —one in fact which might well
demand the expenditure of a million dollars a year and the employment
of a hundred experts of different kinds."[60]

To promote the institute and educate the public to its value, Herty
turned to the press. In February 1919 he gave a lengthy interview to
Edward Marshall, a journalist whose syndicate distributed the interview in newspapers across the United States. Laced with postwar
anti-German propaganda and American boosterism, the interview was

designed to explain to the layman the need for an institute. Herty stressed the empirical nature of existing pharmacology. "How inefficient it is," he exclaimed, "that medicine must take down from the shelf bottle after bottle, trying a dose from each before it finds that which should be administered to the sick in this, the Twentieth Century! . . . Science should be able to predict, in medicine, of all things, not be forced to guess . . . . The situation is so utterly preposterous that it is almost unbelievable."[61] He also praised the Rockefeller Institute but pointed out that it could not accomplish everything alone. Comparing the proposed institute with the Mellon Institute for Industrial Research, Herty said: "The value of the Mellon Institute lies more in the stimulus which it gives to thought and to the desire for industrial chemical research than in the actual results obtained under its roof in the search for valuable secrets of commercial chemistry, and it might well be that a similar comment might after years be made as to the value of such an organization as I suggest for the study of medicinal drugs."

This interview circulated widely and brought further support to the movement. In March 1919 the American Drug Manufacturers Association adopted a resolution supporting the establishment of such an institute. In February 1920, the Medical Sciences Division of the prestigious National Research Council passed a similar resolution.[62] Even more importantly, the interview brought Herty to the attention of Francis P. Garvan, president of the Chemical Foundation. The joining of forces of these two men, coupled with the financial resources of the Chemical Foundation, injected a new dimension of strength into the movement to establish the institute. Their efforts would continue until 1930, when the National Institute of Health became a reality.

Francis Garvan, born June 13, 1875, in East Hartford, Connecticut, was of Irish descent.[63] He was trained as a lawyer and served on the staff of the district attorney of New York City after obtaining his law degree in 1899. When the United States entered World War I, Garvan was made chief of the United States Bureau of Investigation and manager of the New York Office of the Alien Property Custodian. The latter office was charged, among other duties, with breaking up German chemical concerns in the United States, seizing their property, and issuing licenses to American manufacturers for the use of German chemical patents. A. Mitchell Palmer held the office of Alien Property Custodian at this time. As he and Garvan administered their duties, they were appalled by the "extent to which the American chemical industry and related industries . . . were controlled through the medium of international cartel manipulations and foreign owned American patents, the majority of which had been 'shelved' to prevent production in America."[64] Together they hoped to rectify this imbalance. The first German patents captured were sold to American firms, but unregulated sales presented "the probability of an American monopoly through concentration of these patents, and the further possibility of their eventual return to their former [German] owners."[65]

This was unacceptable to Garvan and Palmer, who believed that the captured German patents were of "inestimable value," that they would form the basis for an American synthetic organic chemical industry, and that they would be practically the only compensation the nation would obtain from the war. Thus when Palmer was elevated to attorney general and Garvan succeeded him as alien property custodian, the two argued for the creation of an organization to administer the captured patents equitably. In 1919 they were successful. President Woodrow Wilson organized the Chemical Foundation by executive order, and Garvan became its president.[66]

The private corporation, whose stock was subscribed by the American Dyes Institute, the American Manufacturing Chemists Association, and "other gentlemen engaged in various branches of the chemical industries," issued nonexclusive licenses to American chemical firms for the use of the captured patents.[67] The income derived from this service was used in a variety of ways to promote chemistry in the United States. The Chemical Foundation underwrote the publication costs of several American Chemical Society organs, notably the *Journal of Chemical Education* and *Chemical Abstracts*. It supported the ACS-sponsored high school prize essay contest that was designed to stimulate interest in chemistry among the nation's adolescents. It also published a monograph series in the tradition of Edwin Slosson's popular *Creative Chemistry* and supported the work of numerous university researchers in chemistry.[68]

Shortly after the Chemical Foundation was chartered, Herty wrote an editorial in the *Journal* praising its merits. He did not meet Francis Garvan, however, until after the Edward Marshall interview was published. Impressed by Herty's idea, Garvan invited Herty to his home and offered the financial backing of the Chemical Foundation for promoting public education about the institute. Furthermore, he revealed a personal interest in the undertaking. Garvan's daughter Patricia had died recently "of a streptococcus infection in the blood stream, an incurable disease at the time."[69] Because of this, Garvan and his wife, the former Mabel Brady, had dedicated themselves and their considerable personal wealth to the support of chemistry and medical research.

Garvan offered Herty's committee fifty thousand dollars "to be used in bringing into more definite shape" the plans for the institute.[70] A joint meeting of the committee and representatives of the Chemical Foundation was arranged for October 11, 1920, at the University Club in New York City. As a result of the discussions, a subcommittee was appointed to prepare "a report in popular language of the best means of promoting chemical science for the prevention and cure of disease."[71] This report was to be used "by the officers of the Chemical Foundation in endeavoring to secure a suitable endowment to establish this work on a permanent basis."[72] Members of the subcommittee were Herty as chairman, Reid Hunt, Treat Johnson, Frank Eldred, and Julius Stieglitz.

During the months of discussion about the institute, committee members apparently began to realize that their ultimate goal was broader than the name "Institute for Drug Research" implied. The subcommittee voted unanimously at its meeting on January 15, 1921, to change the name of the committee to "Committee on an Institute for Chemo-Medical Research." The change was approved by the new president of the American Chemical Society, Edgar Fahs Smith.[73]

The broadening of the concept of the institute, the preparation of a document about its mission, and the financial support of the Chemical Foundation increased the possibility that the institute might indeed become a reality. The probability of success, however, was not greeted with universal applause. Intimations of institutional rivalry were perceived by the committee. In December 1919 Herty received a letter from H. Gideon Wells, director of the Otho S. A. Sprague Institute in Chicago. Wells wrote that the Sprague Institute, which had focused on tuberculosis chemotherapy, was considering expanding its concern to chemotherapy in general. Should the proposed institute be established, Wells continued, "it might cause us to modify our plans."[74] Moreover, committee member P. A. Levine distanced himself from the committee during 1920 and finally submitted his resignation that fall. Although Levine claimed that the demands of his work at the Rockefeller Institute prevented further service on the committee, Treat Johnson believed that more serious matters were involved. "I am certain," he wrote Herty, "that the Rockefeller Institute is hostile to organization of competitive institutions."[75] He claimed to have uncovered "certain strong influences which . . . were working against us." What these sinister forces were he did not say. Levine's resignation was accepted, and he was replaced by C. L. Alsberg, chief of the Department of Agriculture's Bureau of Chemistry. Whether active hostility toward the proposed institute actually existed is unclear. There was no further involvement in the committee's work by per-

sonnel of any private institute. Later, when the proposal was under
consideration as a government research facility, representatives from
private institutes heartily endorsed the plan.[76]

When the disturbance over Levine's resignation had abated, the
subcommittee engaged in lively discussion over the emphasis of their
report. Julius Stieglitz wanted to stress the promise of chemotherapy
in medicine. Treat Johnson, in contrast, thought that "the aim of our
institute should be to do that which will lead to an elimination of
drugs."[77] He preferred to emphasize research into fundamental bodily
processes. The final document incorporated both men's interests.
Presented to Francis Garvan August 1, 1921, the report set forth the
basic arguments for cooperative research into fundamental biological
problems and for the development of chemotherapeutic agents. The
operative word throughout was "cooperation." In closing the report,
the committee referred to existing institutions for medical research
and stated:

> There is not a single organization whose purpose is a determined coop-
> erative attack on the problems of disease and health, where intense chem-
> ical and physical research goes hand in hand with the medical and biological
> study of disease. The importance of chemistry and physics has been rec-
> ognized, but the direction of research is still essentially in the hands of
> medical men. No one of the scientific groups alone should be entrusted
> with leadership. All are needed for coping successfully with the complex
> and formidable problems. Complete cooperation of a staff of experts, peers
> in every sense, each in his own field, with emphasis on the fundamental,
> chemical and physical character of the problems, has nowhere been ac-
> complished. Consequently it is proposed that the attack be actually co-
> operative, from the selection of the problem and the formulation of the
> plan of work through the whole concentrated effort to grapple with Nature
> and ultimately to conquer outpost after outpost of the complex world of
> life.[78]

No mention was made in the report, which was published by the
Chemical Foundation in 1921 as *The Future Independence and Progress
of American Medicine in the Age of Chemistry*, of the specific structure
of endowment needed for the proposed institute. Francis Garvan believed that the report "would carry more weight if it were directed to
the general subject of cooperation . . . rather than to be directed
toward the founding of any definite institute."[79] Swayed by Garvan's
opinion, the committee fashioned the report in general terms. The
specific plans drawn up in 1919 were first put into an appendix and
then deleted entirely. It was finally decided that they should be "printed
as a special pamphlet" and distributed to anyone who inquired about

"how the principle involved in the report" could "be best put into actual operation."[80]

The Future Independence and Progress of American Medicine in the Age of Chemistry was widely circulated. Almost 1 million copies were printed at a cost of eighty thousand dollars to the Chemical Foundation. Every physician in the United States received a copy, as did eighty thousand other people, including educators in universities, colleges, and schools; heads of women's organizations; financiers; lawyers; businessmen; Boy Scout masters; editors; agricultural agents; heads of commercial organizations; authors; legislators; public officials; and librarians.[81] The report was well received. Herty notified the committee that a "mass of letters" was "coming in daily."[82]

One response not anticipated was the suggestion that the federal government sponsor the institute. The report had mentioned that of the existing government laboratories, "the Hygienic Laboratory [of the Public Health Service] would be the best adapted for development into a medium of cooperative research."[83] The authors, however, had dismissed this possibility as they had in the past: government salaries could not hold eminent scientists, and the "red tape" involved would stifle creative work. A number of readers of the report disagreed. An editorial review of the document in the *Journal of the American Medical Association* stated that "a government research institute of the type described would be ideal" and suggested that it be located in the Public Health Service.[84]

Albert Widdiss, a circuit judge from Tawas City, Michigan, went even further. Impressed by the report, he gathered signatures on a petition that requested Michigan's Tenth District congressman to introduce into Congress a bill to establish such an institute.[85] Physicist Harvey L. Curtis of the National Bureau of Standards also pressed for government sponsorship. He countered the arguments against federal support, stating that the "opportunity for wide public service is quite as attractive to men as large salaries." As for the money needed to establish an institute, Curtis opined, "If the people of this country are educated to the point where they demand medical research, Congress will be very quick to appropriate the necessary funds."[86]

Committee members were pleased with the favorable response to the report, although Julius Stieglitz and Frank Taylor reemphasized their opposition to government sponsorship. Taylor thought it likely that someone would introduce a bill into Congress; if it happened, he believed that the committee would "have to keep an eye on it and see what the trend of opinion" was.[87] He was correct. In 1924 Senator L. Heisler Ball, a physician from Delaware, introduced a bill to establish a bureau of medical research in the Department of the Interior. There is no record in the correspondence of Herty's committee to indicate that members were aware of the Ball bill. The committee, however, did not hold formal meetings after 1921, so members may well have known about the bill but did not consider it sufficiently viable as to require comment.

Leaders of the Public Health Service, on the other hand, were acutely aware of the Ball bill. They had resisted since the Civil War attempts to establish other medical bureaus that might compete with their leadership in the federal government. Assistant Surgeon General Arthur M. Stimson wrote a memorandum on the bill, S. 3239, in which he stated that it would give rise to "unwarranted and extravagant expenditures in duplication of functions already assigned to the Public Health Service and in particular to the Hygienic Laboratory."[88] Stimson's superior, Secretary of the Treasury Andrew Mellon, wrote to Ball, arguing that the Hygienic Laboratory was indeed carrying on the activities his bill proposed. Quoting from S. 3239, Mellon said:

> At the present time the Public Health Service is conducting at its large and well-appointed Hygienic Laboratory in this city, investigations into "the physical, chemical and biological processes that underlie the functioning of the organs of the human body," is devising "means for controlling the bodily processes" and is determining "the physical, chemical and biological properties of materials when a knowledge of these properties would be of advantage to medical science." I do not contend that this Service is completely covering the enormous field of medical research, but it is, within the limitations imposed by the appropriations, attacking in a rigorously scientific manner pressing problems of physiology and pathology, the solution of which would appear to offer beneficial results in the most fruitful branch of medical science—preventive medicine. The Hygienic Laboratory is provided with an Advisory Board having much the same composition and duties as the proposed Visiting Committee.[89]

Because Senator Ball was not reelected in 1924, his bill did not receive serious consideration. The attempt to establish a medical research bureau in the Interior Department, however, may have contributed to a more favorable response from leaders of the Service to the subsequent National Institute of Health proposal that retained control of medical research in the Public Health Service.

Although the committee did not meet after 1921, Herty submitted yearly reports recommending that the committee be continued. He spoke optimistically about the effects of the published report, even though no funding for the institute had been found. In a handwritten postscript to the 1923 report, Herty noted: "One of the most pronounced effects of our report has been the stimulus to graduate research work in our larger Graduate Schools. I have already experienced its influences here, as many men are writing in to me about biochemistry research. They state in their letters that their interest was stimulated by reading that report."[90] The following year Herty claimed that the report "carried great influence in the determination of the policy pursued by the authorities of both Harvard and Johns Hopkins Universities in their campaigns for funds for their chemistry departments." The University of Wisconsin, moreover, had included "copius extracts" from the committee's report in a brochure that sought funds to establish a National Institute of Research in Colloid Chemistry in Madison. Finally, Georgetown University was "endeavoring to put into practical application a plan for carrying out on a somewhat reduced scale" the principles embodied in the report.[91]

It seemed plain to Herty and other committee members that there was widespread support for a chemo-medical research institute. All that was needed was a benefactor to provide the endowment. Unfortunately, no such philanthropist could be found, and, unlike many other groups seeking funds, neither the Chemical Foundation nor the committee itself seemed to have made a concerted effort to raise the money.[92] There is only one record in the correspondence of the committee relating to a potential donor.[93] In 1926 an attorney in Scranton, Pennsylvania, contacted the president of the American Chemical Society for information about the proposed institute on behalf of an unnamed wealthy client. The letter was referred to Herty, who replied and enclosed a copy of the committee's report. Apparently nothing came of this inquiry; there was no further reference to the matter.

By the mid-1920s there seemed to be little prospect that funding for the proposed institute would materialize. The goal of the committee represented the ideal of cooperation in pure science for the service of mankind, and the approach taken by these men reflected the prevailing conviction about the private sector as the appropriate home for basic research. The lack of a patron for the institute, however, was to make the concept of government funding less noxious as the years passed and the original hope dimmed.

FIVE

Turning to Uncle Sam

I have changed my mind completely,
and I feel that the Government should lead in this matter.
—*Charles Holmes Herty, 1928*

The Great War had permanently enthroned science in American society, but it had not provided a new mechanism for funding the expanded agenda of scientific research. Sentiment remained strong among scientists for private-sector support of their investigations so that highly prized autonomy in research might be maintained. Charles Holmes Herty and other members of the American Chemical Society Committee on an Institute for Chemo-Medical Research continued to believe that with proper publicity for their idea, some wealthy individual would eventually become interested and provide financial backing.

One argument persuading the committee to be patient in seeking a donor was that the inflation and high taxes accompanying World War I had temporarily diminished charitable giving. The sixteenth amendment to the Constitution, which was ratified in 1913 and allowed the taxing of incomes, had been utilized during World War I to raise needed revenues for the war effort. Income rates were raised at every level, reaching 77 percent for personal earnings of $1 million and over.[1] Corporation profits in excess of normal prewar standards were also taxed on a progressive scale. These taxes were lowered somewhat during the postwar years, but they remained high. Secretary of the Treasury Andrew Mellon argued for a drastic reduction in personal taxes during the Harding administration, but Congress held the maximum rate at 50 percent and actually raised the corporate tax from 10 percent to 12.5 percent. With the advent of the Coolidge administration, Congress reduced the maximum rate to 40 percent and in 1926 dropped it even further, to 20 percent.[2] Easing the pinch of high tax rates somewhat were allowable deductions of up to 15 percent for philanthropic giving by individuals. Despite numerous bills to allow similar charitable deductions for corporations, however, none was enacted by Congress until 1936.[3]

It is difficult to assess how severely income taxes affected the ability of wealthy individuals and corporations to make philanthropic contributions for endeavors such as medical research. There was a perception, however, that taxes were a limiting factor. Herty, for instance, wrote to a friend in 1919 about the committee's difficulties in establishing the proposed institute: "Of course, the matter of finance is the main problem now, and it is rendered particularly difficult just at present by the uncertainties of business, pending the signing of the peace treaty and the determination of the policies of the next Congress. To this must of course be added the heavy drain on financial men at present in the form of taxes."[4]

Even though there were pressures from taxation, the number of millionaires in the United States increased throughout the twenties. In 1914 there were an estimated 4,500; by 1926 the figure had grown to 11,000.[5] Given so many potential donors, the argument could perhaps be made that there was no real need for such an institute if patrons were not forthcoming. There was, to be sure, pessimism at this time among some scientists about the likelihood of discovering new chemotherapeutic agents.[6] This lack of progress, however, did not daunt public hopes for new drugs, as the brisk sale of patent medicines demonstrated. The committee had proposed a facility in which basic scientists from a variety of disciplines would work cooperatively and intensively. Could this work have been accomplished in another way? The answer is undoubtedly yes, given a central body such as the National Research Council to coordinate the plans and disperse needed funds. But such a mechanism did not exist in 1919, and, moreover, there was some disagreement in the scientific community over the value of cooperative schemes. Those opposing the idea of cooperation believed that the best hope for scientific discoveries lay with individual scientists laboring alone in their laboratories.[7]

Another possible method for accomplishing the work of the proposed institute would have been to let pharmaceutical firms do the work in their own laboratories. It was commonly agreed that basic research was the long-term key to profits from the application of knowledge; however, the actions of most firms did not support this ideal in fact. Few firms had the financial resources to support in-house basic research on a large scale. Major contributions to university basic science programs would have been an alternative method by which industry could have supported such research, but none except the largest firms chose to commit monies in this way. Indeed, an analysis of the changing patterns of funding for research in the 1920s shows that the Progressive Era equilibrium—private funding for both basic and applied research with a smaller government component for applied work only—was being increasingly destabilized throughout the decade.

Data gathered by the Research Information Service of the National Research Council and published in the *Bulletin of the National Research Council* in 1920, 1928, and 1934 provide virtually the only available information on a nationwide basis about research funds in the private sector during the 1920s.[8] While these data were based on voluntary responses and are occasionally unclear or incomplete, they provide a general picture of how research priorities were changing during the decade of the 1920s. These funds came from private individuals, professional associations, honorary societies, and occasionally from individual businesses. The bulk of the funds was expended in universities. Private-sector expenditures for scientific research of all types, including medicine, rose from $5,285,245 in 1920 to $14,421,403 in 1928. The effect of the Great Depression is clearly visible in the 1934 figure: it remained nearly static at $14,723,673, an absolute increase of only 2.1 percent over the 1928 amount.

The most dramatic change that occurred during this period was in the amounts designated for research on applied subjects. Funds designated for industrial research were only 1.62 percent of the total in 1920. By 1928 they had jumped to 9.18 percent of all funds expended for scientific research. This pattern was repeated to an even greater degree in agricultural research. In 1920 agricultural research made up 3.73 percent of the total; in 1928 this jumped to 21.72 percent.

Basic scientific disciplines—chemistry, physics, and biology—in which much basic research relating to medicine occurred, suffered in relation to applied fields. Funds for research in biology, for example, declined from 11.92 percent of the total in 1920 to 10.74 percent of the total in 1928. Funds for physics, likewise, decreased from 7.20 percent of the total to 4.24 percent of the total during this period.

Funds in all of these disciplines increased absolutely during the 1920s, but applied fields were clearly the areas in which researchers could expect generous support. Most of the funds for industrial and agricultural research were donated by professional associations representing businesses in some particular field of endeavor. In Illinois, for example, the Illinois Canning Association made $2,700 per year available for "sweet corn investigation."[9] Individual firms did contribute to research, but their numbers were small. Of 903 individual funds for research—excluding prizes, medals, and fellowships—only 43 were donated by individual businesses over the fourteen-year period.[10] Many of these firms, moreover, were the leaders of their field with a more comfortable profit margin than their less well-known competitors. The Kellogg cereal company, the Firestone rubber company, the DuPont rayon company, and the Fleischmann yeast company were some of the firms that contributed more than $1,000 a year to research in universities. Nearly all of these contributions were designated for highly specific investigations rather than for basic research.

Industry, then, was hardly a promising source of support for the kind of pure chemo-medical research proposed by the ACS committee. The trend of support for medical research in general during the 1920s was also toward increasing the level of applied research to the detriment of basic investigations. In 1920 funding for "general medical research" and for broad areas such as anatomy, physiology, and pathology constituted 83 percent of all medical funds reported by the National Research Council. By 1928 this had decreased to 78.83 percent while funds for categorical research on specific diseases had increased. There were twenty-four categories for which funds were designated in 1920; this number had more than doubled by 1928, to fifty.[11] New funds, most of which were for relatively small amounts of money, were established for special studies on problems such as the "common cold" and "nervous disease."

Whether the donor was a private citizen or a philanthropic foundation, the increasing tendency to fund categorical research prevailed. The Rockefeller Foundation, for example, determined in 1928 to reorient its giving policies so that they would be more relevant to human problems.[12] This did not necessarily mean that basic sciences would be cut off but that their role was to be viewed as contributory to areas more easily understood by the public as practical.

One of the major reasons the Rockefeller and other private foundations began to focus their monies toward particular projects was the escalating demands made upon them during the 1920s. College enrollments boomed after World War I. Between 1900 and 1930 the percentage of the population between the ages of eighteen and twenty-one enrolled in institutions of higher education increased from 4 percent to 12.42 percent.[13] In the five-year period from 1923 to 1928 alone, enrollment at 216 colleges and universities on the approved list of the Association of American Universities jumped 25 percent.[14] Colleges responded to this acceleration by hiring more instructors and building more dormitories and classroom buildings. Much of the cost of increasing the size of physical plants was borne by foundations, especially for new science buildings. In addition to donations for bricks and mortar, foundations were committed to supporting fellowships in universities.[15] The sciences were popular subjects after World War I; with a steadily increasing number of industrial laboratories in the

1920s, graduates with degrees in science could look forward confidently to employment.[16]

Increasing pressure for funds in all areas and the trend toward funding applied or categorical projects helped to discourage philanthropists and foundations from considering proposals for the establishment of new institutes such as the one Herty and his associates wanted. This situation existed at the same time that scientific research and scientific medicine were becoming identified in the public's mind as the source of a better life. The labor-saving devices and other technological innovations that appeared in the 1920s were perceived by the public to be the fruits of scientific research, and a continued stream of new inventions was confidently expected. Such an attitude, however, was to some extent a double-edged sword for the scientific community. Lafayette B. Mendel, professor of chemistry at Yale University, observed in 1927: "The word research has become an expression to conjure with; a term used not infrequently without any adequate appreciation of its fundamental implications. Thus it has come about that science has been exposed upon an elevated pedestal to the fullest view of an over-awed public."[17]

Mendel was concerned about the public's tendency to assume that "a little enthusiasm and well directed energy will inevitably furnish the required solutions" to mankind's problems. And yet scientists themselves were inclined to an optimism about the promise of science that bordered on determinism. From World War I through the 1920s the more speculative articles in *Science* were laced with this sort of positivism.[18]

Popular magazines reflected a similar tone, but they focused primarily on applied science. There was, in fact, a marked shift from 1900 to 1930 in the percentages of magazine articles devoted to basic and applied topics. According to the 1933 report of the President's Commission on Social Trends, the number of articles per thousand indexed on basic subjects dropped from 12.75 in 1900 to 7.29 in 1930, a decrease of 43 percent. During this same period, the number of articles on applied subjects rose from 0.88 to 6.73, an increase of 664 percent.[19]

Medical research was classified as applied research in the commission's study; hence it enjoyed rising popularity in the 1920s. It was not research alone, however, that had captured the public's confidence. The medical profession had achieved what Paul Starr has described as "cultural authority," a status of respect and trust it had not enjoyed during most of the nineteenth century. Starr traced this phenomenon both to the power of scientific medicine to cure some infectious diseases and to urbanization and industrialization in the United

States, which radically altered the traditional nineteenth-century way of life.[20] Leaders in both the medical and public health fields took advantage of this high public regard to disseminate the gospel of personal hygiene and scientific medicine throughout the country. The art of public relations, which was rapidly developing in the 1920s, assisted them in this effort. The American Medical Association, for example, began publication of its popular health magazine *Hygeia* in 1923, filling it with timely articles on personal health, answers to readers' health questions, and special sections for children such as songs and poems promoting the value of sunshine and milk. The American Public Health Association, which likewise began in 1919 the publication of a popular health magazine, *The Nation's Health*, also established a special section on public health education. Writers for this section's column in the association's official organ, the *American Journal of Public Health*, discussed the organization of local health education campaigns, proposed slogans, and even provided detailed advice on how to format brochures to capture a reader's attention.

The result of such efforts was a growth of positive feeling for public health measures, scientific medicine, and scientific research. The messages quickly permeated the fabric of American life. Robert and Helen Lynd reported in their classic study *Middletown* that by 1924 courses in hygiene and health were routinely included in the elementary school curriculum, a situation that had not existed in 1890. Furthermore, the kinds of questions asked of school children in 1890 had given way by 1924 to those tinged with an acceptance of the authority of scientific medicine. The Lynds observed: "Characteristic questions of 1890 such as 'Describe each of the two kinds of matter of the nervous system' and 'Tell weight and shape of the brain. Tell names of membranes around it.' are being replaced by 'Write a paragraph describing exactly the kind of shoe you should wear, stating all the good points and the reasons for them,' and 'What is the law of muscles and bones (regarding posture)? How should you guide your daily life?' "[21]

For adults there were magazine articles and books with advice on weight control, exercise, ventilation, sleep habits, and other health concerns. Irving Fisher, whose 1909 *Report on National Vitality* had helped spark the campaign for a national department of health, joined with Eugene Lyman Fisk of the Life Extension Institute to publish a book in 1915 that brought together much of this sort of advice. Boldly entitled *How to Live*, the book went through eighteen editions by 1926.[22] The public was clearly hungry for information and hopeful that medical science would continue to provide preventive advice and to develop new therapies for the ills of mankind.

These characteristics of the 1920s—confidence in science, scientific medicine, and public health; a positivistic outlook within the scientific community; a rapid rise in college enrollments and in the number of scientists; pressure on the resources of foundations and philanthropists; and increasing emphasis on applied research—all exerted pressure to destabilize the accepted allocation of responsiblity for the funding of scientific research of all types. The assumption that basic research was appropriately the province of the private sector alone while applied research would be pursued by both the government and the private sector was reaching the limits of what was financially possible.

Attitudes did not quickly change about the division of responsibility, however. As was previously mentioned, throughout the early 1920s, the members of the Committee on an Institute for Chemo-Medical Research continued to envision their proposed institute as a private-sector enterprise. Other scientists likewise sought greater support from the private sector to finance an expansion of research. In 1925 the National Academy of Sciences inaugurated a campaign to raise funds from industry for the support of university research in pure science. The National Research Fund, as it was called, was chaired by then Secretary of Commerce Herbert Hoover and promoted vigorously by George Ellery Hale. The fund failed to receive widespread support from industry, and by 1932, given the death blow by the Depression, it expired. Lance E. Davis and Daniel J. Kevles have argued that such a fund would probably have failed even without the intervention of the economic crisis, because businesses were reluctant to contribute to basic science research from which they could reap no exclusive profits. [23] The patterns of giving to university research reported by the National Research Council would seem to provide additional evidence in support of this contention.

In the physical and biological sciences, the problem of funding for basic research was not resolved until after World War II when the National Science Foundation was established. [24] With regard to basic biomedical research, however, events took a different course that opened the federal purse sooner for pure science, at least to a limited extent.

The chairman of the ACS Committee on an Institute for Chemo-Medical Research, Charles Holmes Herty, spent the years from 1921 to 1926 as president of the newly created Synthetic Organic Chemical Manufacturers Association (SOCMA). Having been associated with the Allied commission after World War I in negotiating for the United States' share of German reparation dyes, Herty had gained a reputation as a champion of the emerging American synthetic organic chemical industry. As president of SOCMA he continued to promote "chemical independence" for American firms until 1926, when he resigned to become a scientific advisor to the Chemical Foundation. These five years of lobbying on behalf of the chemical industry acquainted Herty with the subtleties of the congressional process and increased his understanding of how effectively federal support could advance a favored cause.

It was perhaps this experience that by 1926 made Herty at least willing to entertain the idea of government sponsorship for the proposed institute. While visiting in Washington, D.C., in January 1926, he had an "interesting talk" with Louisiana senator Joseph Eugene Ransdell.[25] Herty provided Ransdell, who was "deeply interested in the possibilities of chemistry in the alleviation of suffering," with a copy of *The Future Independence and Progress of American Medicine in the Age of Chemistry* and a report on the newly established Boyce Thompson Institute for Plant Research. Hoping for Ransdell's endorsement, Herty followed up their meeting with a letter to Ransdell in which he implored, "Whatever you might find yourself in a position to do to bring this thought home to our people will certainly be a lasting contribution to a cause which all lovers of humanity have deep at heart."[26] Ransdell, having read the committee's report, replied a month later. "The more I think about your proposition of establishing a great research laboratory to study all diseases of human beings," he said, "the more impressed I am by its wisdom."[27]

In mid-March the two men met again. Over lunch Ransdell spoke "of his desire to help the matter forward in some way."[28] Herty suggested that Ransdell make a speech on the floor of the Senate, but Ransdell wanted "something definite" about which to speak. Ransdell proposed that he draft a bill to create the institute as a government undertaking, that he ask for hearings, and that he speak in support of his bill. Herty was pleased with Ransdell's interest, but "told him frankly" that the committee preferred private-sector sponsorship. He promised, however, to consult committee members immediately about Ransdell's proposal.

The responses Herty received to his inquiry about Ransdell's sponsorship of a bill fell into three groups. Treat Johnson and F. O. Taylor opposed any government involvement. "Our institute," Johnson wrote, "must be a privately endowed organization."[29] Taylor concurred, believing that favorable public opinion for the institute, "especially in the minds of those who may eventually be able to finance so great an undertaking, is slowly developing and will be the sounder for its slow growth."[30] He feared that a "big project that grows too rapidly is more likely to possess more of the characteristics of the mushroom than the oak." Raymond Bacon and John J. Abel took a moderate position on Ransdell's advocacy. "It would be my feeling," Bacon wrote, ". . . that the publicity thus obtained could not possibly hurt our situation and might be a great help."[31] Reid Hunt, Julius Stieglitz, and Carl Alsberg were even more positive. Stieglitz believed Ransdell should be encouraged, and he stated pragmatically, "Any research institution with adequate financial support would be better than none."[32] Hunt and Alsberg, both of whom had previously held positions in government laboratories, suggested that the Public Health Service was the logical place for such work. Alsberg pointed out that "some of the most notable achievements in the field of chemo-therapy have been produced in government research institutes."[33] He cited Paul Ehrlich's Imperial Institute for Therapeutic Research and "the work in chemo-therapy of the [Interdepartmental] Social Hygiene Board, much of which was excellent and which was formerly supported by Federal funds." With a positive response from five of his seven committee members, Herty advised Ransdell to proceed.

Joseph Eugene Ransdell, a stocky Southern gentleman with a goatee, was to succeed in creating what he chose to call the National Institute of Health where all previous efforts, public and private, had failed. Born October 7, 1858, Ransdell was the son of a newspaper editor who later turned to farming.[34] Ransdell's father, John H. Ransdell, was killed in a farm accident in 1869, and his mother, Amanda Louise Terrell Ransdell, was left with nine children to rear. At age nineteen, Ransdell, the next to youngest in the devout Roman Catholic family, won a scholarship to Union College in Schenectady, New York. After his graduation in 1882, he studied law privately and was admitted to the Louisiana bar in 1883. He was elected district attorney in Lake Providence, Louisiana in 1884, an office he held for twelve years. In 1899 he won a seat in Congress from Louisiana's Fifth Congressional District. While in the House of Representatives, Ransdell sat on the Rivers and Harbors Committee, and he was influential in organizing the National Rivers and Harbors Congress in 1906. He served as head of this body for fourteen years. Ransdell also visited Panama at the time the Panama Canal was being constructed. There he met William Gorgas and discussed with him the efforts made to eradicate malaria and yellow fever from the Canal Zone.[35]

After winning a seat in the United States Senate in 1912, Ransdell broadened his interest to include health legislation. As chairman of the Senate Committee on Public Health, he made a speech in 1916 entitled "Rural Health, the Nation's First Duty." In this speech Ransdell adopted two themes of the national health movement that later appeared in his efforts to establish the National Institute of Health. The first was to emphasize the economy of preventive medicine over therapeutic treatment, an idea popularized by Irving Fisher in his 1909 *Report on National Vitality.* The second was to stress federal responsibility in public health matters, an argument he based on the fact that "disease has absolutely no regard for state lines."[36]

Ransdell also made a comprehensive study of leprosy in the United States during his tenure as chairman of the Public Health Committee. This led him to introduce legislation for the federal government to take over the existing Louisiana Home for Lepers at Carville. The leprosarium, established in 1894, had already been considered for purchase by the Public Health Service, which was seeking a treatment center for leprosy patients. It had been rejected, however, because of its distance from a major medical center and what was believed to be an unhealthy climate.[37] Other states, unfortunately, did not want a leprosarium within their boundaries; hence the Louisiana Home for Lepers was finally selected by default. Ransdell's legislation creating the National Leprosarium was signed into law by Woodrow Wilson on February 3, 1917, and the Public Health Service assumed control in 1921.

By 1926 Ransdell had been in Congress for twenty-seven years, longer than any other Louisiana congressman. Perhaps the greatest lesson he had learned in his many legislative battles was that persistence and compromise were the keys to success. His advocacy of the National Institute of Health would require four years and many compromises. Throughout that time his enthusiasm never flagged, and his persistence was well known. In 1927 Surgeon General Cumming expressed the wish that Ransdell had been the sponsor of the Parker bill to reorganize the Service and coordinate federal health activities "because of his pushing ability and enthusiasm."[38]

In April 1926 Ransdell's enthusiasm for the proposed institute was first put to the test. Knowing that any bill he introduced would be referred to the Senate Commerce Committee, Ransdell polled that body for opinions on the proposed institute. He found them "at wide variance" on the idea. Writing to Herty, he said, "Some of the members think it would be a good thing to have such a bill introduced. Others feel that it is not advisable, while a third element feels that the important work now being done by the United States Public Health Service should be better supported and far greater facilities provided."[39]

In the face of the questionable reception from the Commerce Committee, Herty suggested moving in another direction. He was aware that the Public Health Service was promoting the Parker bill, which included a provision for expanding the Hygienic Laboratory, and he believed that the chemo-medical research institute might appropriately

be included in an expanded version of the bill. He suggested that
Ransdell introduce the Parker bill into the Senate. "It seems to me,"
he wrote Ransdell, "there is just the opportunity for the expansion of
this work along the lines suggested in our report, and a discussion of
that on the floor of the Senate would give most valuable publicity."[40]
At this time Ransdell did not act on Herty's suggestion. Ransdell did
make contact with leaders of the Public Health Service, and he found
them at best lukewarm about his proposed legislation. He wrote Herty:
"I find that the chiefs of this service would like very much to have
additional funds, but they have been intimidated against asking for
same by the stringent rules of the Budget, hence they are averse to
the introduction of any bill which looks to greater appropriation for
their work."[41]

Indeed, neither Ransdell nor any member of Herty's committee
actually believed that the Budget Bureau or its formidable chief Herbert M. Lord would approve an appropriation to create the institute.
Nonetheless, Ransdell collaborated with Assistant Surgeon General
John W. Kerr of the Public Health Service in drafting a bill that incorporated some Service goals with Ransdell's National Institute of
Health proposal.[42] Having decided to go ahead with the idea in spite
of the odds against passage, Ransdell introduced his bill as S. 4540
on July 1, 1926.[43] He apparently decided upon the name "National
Institute of Health" at the last minute. A typescript of the speech he
delivered July 2 in support of the bill shows clearly an erasure and the
insertion of the chosen name.[44] Quoting extensively from *The Future
Independence and Progress of American Medicine in the Age of Chemistry*, Ransdell laid before the Senate the major arguments in favor of
creating the institute—the high cost of sickness, the lack of cooperation among existing institutions in America, the need for federal
leadership in combatting a problem that crossed state lines. "Under
the Constitution," he said,

> scientific research is a fundamental function of the Federal Government
> . . . . The promotion of scientific research by means of special appropri-
> ations to maintain laboratories has been the policy followed by our Federal
> Government and many state governments. Thus far the field covered has
> been limited . . . . The system of maintenance of research by means of
> appropriations should be continued. In future, the effort should be to utilize
> these appropriations not only for the conduct of investigations but the
> coordination of scientific effort and the maintenance of advisory and su-
> pervisory agents in the interest of science.[45]

The bill itself provided for the establishment of a National Institute
of Health in the Public Health Service. Its connection to the existing

Hygienic Laboratory was not specified in the text of the bill, but Ransdell clearly believed that the Institute would supersede the Laboratory. In his speech he had noted that the "present Hygienic Laboratory is a fine start. Its buildings are small but its work has been magnificent. Why not make it the nucleus of the great institution outlined above?"[46] The bill carried an appropriation of $5 million for the selection of a site and construction of necessary buildings. An additional $2 million per year for five years was to be used to enlarge the Hygienic Laboratory and to establish fellowships "to bestow upon scientists of proven proficiency in researches affecting public health." Fellowships were mentioned again in a section of the bill authorizing the secretary of the Treasury to accept private contributions to the Institute. Any donations received were to be used "for study, investigation, and research in pure science," and fellowships were one specific item designated as an appropriate means to further this goal. Contributions of $500,000 or more would bear the name of the donor. The proposed fellowships were modeled on the industrial fellowships of the Mellon Institute and were intended for working scientists, not for students.

Fellows, as well as resident Public Health Service researchers, could elect, under another provision of the bill, to pursue a course of study prescribed by the Surgeon General and receive a graduate degree, presumably in public health. Such a graduate program had been suggested by the Service since 1907.[47] In the appointment of personnel, Institute staff members would be exempt from the Classification Act of 1923 that restricted the salaries of scientists who were not physicians. Finally, the facilities of the Institute were to be extended to state and local health authorities when needed, another longstanding Service goal that had been followed for years in practice but never incorporated into law.

The appropriation for the proposed National Institute of Health closely paralleled the amount projected in 1919 by the Committee on an Institute for Chemo-Medical Research as necessary to establish and maintain a research facility. The committee had estimated a total endowment of $10.4 million; Ransdell's bill provided $15 million over five years. The provision for exempting scientists from the restrictive Civil Service classification system was also derived from the committee's desire to secure the best scientific minds. Under existing Civil Service salaries, many scientists would not have been interested.

The proposal for private donations to fund fellowships at the Institute reveals best the change that had occurred in the thinking of Herty and his fellow committee members. Such a fellowship provision remained constant in all versions of the bill throughout its years before

Congress and was stressed in every hearing and floor debate. Herty, Ransdell, and other proponents of the bill clearly expected large private donations to flow into the Institute, once established. Because of this, it seems likely that these men were not changing their philosophy radically with regard to public and private support of research. Herty testified at hearings on the bill in 1928 that although as chairman of the ACS committee he had championed the creation of a private-sector institute, "I have changed my mind completely, and I feel that the Government should lead in this matter."[48] The government's leadership, it was proposed, would be supplemented generously by private donations. This position was similar to that of Herbert Hoover, who as secretary of Commerce believed that government should be used to stimulate private-sector participation in what Ellis W. Hawley has called the "associative state."[49] These men continued to support the ideals of American individualism and were generally cool, if not hostile, to the strong social action programs proposed later during the New Deal. Government leadership for an enterprise that was expected to receive private-sector support, however, was a different matter in this view.

Shortly after the Ransdell bill was introduced, it received an endorsement from the *New York Times*. Drawing its arguments largely from the heritage of the public health and conservation movements, the editorial stated:

> Research service in the conservation of the health of the nation should not be left entirely to private interest, however generous, zealous, and intelligent. Particularly it is desirable that chemistry should be brought back, in its highest development as a science, to the aid of the physician in the prevention of disease and the alleviation of suffering. It has turned its attention in recent decades mainly to the production of wealth in the industries. It has a higher ministry before it if it can be brought to cope with disease in time of peace as its aid was invoked by the Government during the war. We have gone further in our Federal departments in concern for the health of lower animals, and even of trees and plants, than we have for that of human beings.[50]

This editorial demonstrates how the old arguments had been transferred from a national department of health proposal to a plan for expanded scientific research in health-related fields. World War I had stimulated this new awareness of science as a potential force for service to mankind. The older goal of establishing a coordinated federal health department was still alive in the form of the Parker bill, but its rhetoric now had to be shared with the strong claim for better health through research represented by the proposal for a National Institute of Health.

As the first session of the Sixty-Ninth Congress ended, both the Ransdell and Parker bills were lodged in committee. During the next four years the proponents of both bills engaged in what might best be described in musical terms as a counterpoint figure with supporters of the other bill. Like a two-voice fugue, they were occasionally in competition with one another, while at other times they reinforced each other's efforts. Fortunately, as the years passed, the political climate improved so that their chances for success were significantly greater than those of their Progressive Era counterparts.

PART THREE

Creating a National Institute of Health, 1926–1937

SIX

Vision and Reality in New Era Politics

I do not believe that permanency of appointment of those engaged in
the professional and scientific activities of the Government
is necessary for progress or accomplishment in those
activities or in keeping with public policy.
—*Calvin Coolidge, 1928*

In 1926 Calvin Coolidge was presiding over unprecedented prosperity in the United States. The stock market climbed, modern technology provided a seemingly ever-increasing stream of devices to make life more pleasant, and there was a wide-spread optimism that America would continue to grow and prosper indefinitely. Coolidge's approach to governing an expanding economy was to minimize the role of government and encourage private-sector initiative. Herbert M. Lord, director of the Bureau of the Budget, rigidly enforced Coolidge's economy program within the government. Proposals for the expansion of existing bureaus or the creation of new ones were generally opposed during the New Era. There were exceptions, of course. The Commerce Department expanded under its secretary, Herbert Hoover, and some programs relating to military interest, such as the Veterans' Bureau, continued to flourish. These special concerns of the Coolidge administration, however, underscored its overall commitment to private business and the necessity of responding to powerful lobbies.

Coolidge did not believe in marked expansion of governmental intitatives to promote health. He frequently lauded the medical profession and acclaimed scientists for their contribution to the national weal, but he viewed medicine and science as appropriately the province of the private sector. He addressed the American Medical Association (AMA) at its 1927 annual meeting, for example, conferring "high praise" on the association for its "contribution to American medicine."[1] In his 1924 book, *The Price of Freedom*, Coolidge also wrote that "the world today is absolutely dependent on science and commerce."[2] He was willing to enforce Progressive Era health regulatory legislation and to

extend it to a limited degree. He approved, for instance, the Federal
Caustic Poison Bill in 1927 that required "household packages of lye,
ammonia, carbolic acid, oxalic acid, and other caustic substances . . .
to be distinctly labeled 'Poison,' with instructions as to emergency
treatment in case of accident."[3]

Such regulatory legislation, however, was circumscribed and did
not address the larger problems of curing disease and promoting public
health measures. Whereas Hermann M. Biggs took as the motto of
the *New York State Department of Health Bulletin*: "Public Health is
Purchasable. Within Natural Limitations Any Community Can Determine Its Own Death Rate," Coolidge rejected the notion that the
welfare of the citizenry—which included its health—was related to
economics.[4] He stated in 1921:

> The question of human welfare is not an economic question. It is a moral
> question. There is no difficulty with the present advance of scientific knowl-
> edge in providing for the welfare of the race. The ability is not lacking
> even if no further advance were made in discovery and invention. The
> material and intellectual force are sufficient. They could be much greater—
> must be made much greater, but the present deficiency is not there. It
> is the disposition—the moral force that is lacking. Men are not doing as
> well as they can with what they have.[5]

In this speech Coolidge was addressing the larger question of public
welfare. Such an attitude, however, did not dispose him favorably
toward the encouragement of greater federal involvement in health
matters. His philosophy toward public health is perhaps best revealed
in what he did not say rather than in any overt opposition to health
legislation. As president, Coolidge never mentioned public health specifically in any of his speeches.

It was during this conservative administration that the Ransdell and
Parker bills were introduced. The Parker bill, representing the allied
goals of the Public Health Service and the national health movement,
sought approval for reorganizing the Service to reflect the growth that
the agency had undergone since 1912. It proposed consolidation of
other federal health agencies of the government with the Service to
secure a more efficient federal health program. It also contained modest provisions for expanding research in the Hygienic Laboratory and
elevating the status and compensation of many Service personnel. In
short, the Parker bill was written to achieve as much as possible within
the clearly understood limits of the Coolidge philosophy of limited
government.

Senator Ransdell's bill for a National Institute of Health, in contrast,
boldly proposed a large expenditure for the creation of a new agency

that would expand federal activity in medical research to include basic investigations as well as vigorously prosecuted applied research. Originated and supported by members of the scientific research community, this bill embodied the confidence of science and virtually ignored political realities.

Because the approaches taken to these two proposals were so different, there were bound to be difficulties as the proponents of each bill attempted to work together in the legislative process. This first became clear in the fall of 1926, when the supporters of the Ransdell bill attempted to get national publicity for the idea of a research institute. Francis Garvan, president of the Chemical Foundation, had decided to support the bill as the most likely way to implement the research program outlined by the American Chemical Society (ACS) Committee for an Institute on Chemo-Medical Research. Through the Chemical Foundation, Garvan provided financial support and authorized Charles Holmes Herty, who had become a full-time scientific advisor to the Foundation in 1926, to work closely with Senator Ransdell in the effort to get the bill passed.

One of Herty's first actions was to publish on the editorial page of the Sunday *New York Times* an article calling for "a national campaign sponsored and financed by the United States government against disease."[6] He suggested that a national convention be held in Washington, D.C., shortly after the new Congress convened to "show the sentiment in this country in favor of public health."[7] Senator Ransdell, Herty, and representatives of the Public Health Service met in August to discuss this idea. Surgeon General Hugh Cumming believed the proposed conference to be "a rather doubtful expedient."[8] He wrote to Ransdell that it would seem "wise to defer making any definite plans regarding this matter until it has been discussed with the leaders in the public health movements."[9]

In early November Ransdell again talked with leaders of the Service. Again they temporized. Ransdell wrote to Herty that "General Cumming seemed intensely interested, just as he did before, but I read between the lines of his talk that he is skittish about the Budget Officer."[10] Similar negotiations dragged on for another month before the plan for the conference was abandoned. By that time it was clear to Ransdell and Herty that Public Health Service leaders did not share their sweeping vision of a national health research institute.

The Surgeon General and his top advisors actually had mixed feelings about Ransdell's proposal. Cumming and Assistant Surgeon General John Kerr, who had assisted Ransdell in drafting the National Institute of Health bill, favored the bill's goal of increasing research facilities. They were, however, skeptical about the Budget Bureau's approval of the large appropriation the bill carried.[11] Three crucial Service leaders, furthermore, were not enthusiastic about the bill. George W. McCoy, director of the Hygienic Laboratory; Rolla Eugene Dyer, assistant director of the Hygienic Laboratory; and Arthur M. Stimson, director of the Division of Scientific Research, "could not visualize with Ransdell a quantum jump in size and activity of research."[12] Stimson asserted: "It is believed to be a good principle that the growth of government services is most calculated to serve the people best when it is evolutionary in nature." He questioned, quite legitimately, whether the Hygienic Laboratory could make adequate use of such large amounts of money as the bill proposed in such a short time. "It is believed," he continued, "that the sudden quadrupling or more of such funds would not result in proportionate output. An attempt at such rapid expansion would result, it is believed, in wasteful methods, confusion of purpose and the ill considered employment of personnel. A better course is believed to be found in the gradual expansion as need is evident and as personnel is available."[13]

Rolla E. Dyer, who was to serve as director of the National Institute of Health from 1942 until 1950 during a period of rapid expansion in which three new institutes were added to the facility and its name made plural, was not convinced in 1926 that Ransdell's plan had much merit. He, too, believed that "the expansion of the Laboratory . . . should be considered in the light of a slow or deliberate growth rather than growth of a mushroom type." Moreover, Dyer counseled caution regarding the provision of the Ransdell bill that allowed private contributions for research. He opposed perpetuating the names of donors who gave large amounts and believed the actual probability that such gifts would be offered to be remote.[14]

George McCoy, ten-year veteran director of the Hygienic Laboratory, believed that the provision allowing private gifts was "rather humiliating for the government," because it suggested that Uncle Sam was "unable or unwilling to support necessary public health research." He also believed that the Ransdell bill intended "to appropriate the record of creditable service of the Hygienic Laboratory and the prestige attaching to it" for the new National Institute of Health.[15]

Discussions between Ransdell and the Public Health Service apparently led to consideration that the Ransdell and Parker bills might be combined, for early in January 1927 Treasury Secretary Andrew Mellon proposed exactly that in a letter to Senator Wesley Jones, chairman of the Committee on Commerce. He warned that an appropriations increase would hinder passage, although, he said, "this, of course, would not apply to private bequests."[16] Less than three weeks later an analysis of the Ransdell bill made by a staff member in the Budget Bureau recommended combining the two bills. As the memorandum went up the bureacratic ladder, however, the original recommendation was reversed. Charles H. Fullaway, assistant to the director of the Budget, penciled a handwritten explanation of his change of mind, concluding with the observation that "the proposals in the attached bill are unreasonable."[17]

Unaware of the opposition of the Budget Bureau, Ransdell, Herty, and the Surgeon General discussed the possible merger of the bills over lunch in February. Cumming, Herty perceived, was much more interested in the Parker bill than in Ransdell's proposed expansion of research. Nonetheless, "I fanned the flame of union," Herty reported to Francis Garvan at the Chemical Foundation.[18] "I think," he went on, that "the whole subject is now taking a very healthy direction."

Herty's optimism was short-lived. Assistant Surgeon General John Kerr drafted the combined bill, which was introduced as S. 5835 on March 2, 1927. In a subsequent memorandum to Garvan, Herty expressed his reservations:

> [Ransdell] agreed with me that the combined Ransdell-Parker bill, as drawn up by Dr. Kerr . . . was a plain case of the tail wagging the dog—many important features of the original bill have been omitted. From the discussion it was soon evident that neither General Cumming nor Dr. Kerr had been able to grasp the possibility of securing from Congress anything more that the meager appropriations they have been receiving in the past, nor had they stopped to think what might be accomplished with aroused public sentiment.[19]

The new bill contained all the features of the original Parker bill, incorporated portions of the Ransdell bill, and designated a $10 million appropriation for the proposed institute.[20] Considering the existing opposition of the Budget Bureau to Ransdell's proposal, it came as no surprise that the new bill was not approved by that agency.

Surgeon General Cumming's preoccupation with the Parker bill was understandable. Hearings on the House version of the bill, which did not contain the National Institute of Health proposal, were scheduled before a subcommittee of the House Interstate and Foreign Commerce Committee February 24 and 25. Convincing the committee to report the bill favorably would be a difficult task, because President Coolidge, according to Budget Director Lord, still objected to the sections of the bill that offered commissions to nonmedical personnel, raised Service officers to ranks comparable with those of the military, and created a nurse corps.[21] Lord claimed that the president suggested the introduction of a substitute bill without these so-called military provisions. Service leaders, however, hoped to secure passage with the disputed provisions intact.[22]

In mid-January 1927, Haley Fiske, president of the Metropolitan Life Insurance Company and member of the National Health Council, came to Washington to confer with Service leaders about the legislation. Surgeon General Cumming and John Kerr met Fiske at the train station, and on their way to the Washington Hotel, the three discussed Coolidge's objections.[23] They all agreed that the personnel provisions were "the heart of the bill." Kerr, therefore, began to prepare lists of potential witnesses who could testify in favor of these sections.[24] Final strategy was planned with several of the witnesses over breakfast at the Cosmos Club the morning of the hearings.[25]

Testimony was carefully orchestrated to be favorable to the bill. Surprisingly, it was not the personnel provisions that drew criticism from a few witnesses but rather section one—the National Health Council–sponsored provision to transfer other federal agencies into the Public Health Service. National Health Council representatives James A. Tobey and Donald Armstrong made the case for consolidation. Armstrong explained the rationale of the groups that had sponsored the bill.[26] Tobey summarized the main points he had made in *The National Government and Public Health* and offered to supply each committee member with a copy of the book.[27] Further, he emphasized the number of different nongovernmental health agencies that had endorsed that bill. "The bill is a joint effort," he said, and "is the first time that the public health profession and the medical profession and the industrial organizations concerned with health and political scientists and everybody else interested in the subject have united on a bill that they are all agreed on is effective and if enacted will be efficacious."[28]

Unfortunately for Tobey, he was not correct in asserting complete unanimity for the plan. Representatives of other organizations endorsed the idea of cooperation, but many had reservations about the crucial first section. Edgar Wallace, representing the American Federation of Labor, objected to the power given the executive department to transfer agencies.[29] He preferred to entrust that power to Congress. William C. Fowler, health officer of the District of Columbia, feared that the health department of the District might be separated from the municipal government under section one.[30] These and other speakers urged coordination but requested a reconsideration of consolidation.

In his remarks to the subcommittee, Surgeon General Cumming gingerly avoided giving wholehearted support to section one. Instead he emphasized section two, which allowed the detailing of Service officers to other bureaus. William H. Welch, seventy-seven years old and one of the most respected figures in American medicine, supported Cumming. It must have been "forty years ago at least," he said, recalling his involvement in a national health department campaign of the late 1890s,

> that I accompanied a delegation from the New York Academy of Medicine in support of a bill to create a Federal department of health. I have long since ceased to feel any interest in efforts to create . . . a separate department of health. . . . I think the second part [of the Parker bill] . . . is possibly more important, namely, the definite authorization of the detail of medical officers, scientists, and experts from the Public Health Service to the various bureaus and departments.[31]

Welch waxed most eloquent when he addressed the subject of medical research in the Hygienic Laboratory. He encouraged the committee to approve the sections of the bill allowing exchanges of personnel with universities for research purposes and providing for expansion of the number of divisions in the Hygienic Laboratory. "I do not think our country is fully alive," he observed, "to what scientific research means for the advancement of the civilization of the country and for the welfare of the people."[32]

Milton J. Rosenau, former director of the Hygienic Laboratory, also spoke strongly for these provisions. "I believe we can put it down almost as an axiom," he said, "that our ability to control any disease is just about directly proportional to our knowledge of that disease. . . . The only way to find out more about such diseases is to study them—in the laboratory, in the field, at the bedside—by the methods of science. Those who are willing to devote themselves to such work should be given adequate facilities for the work."[33] Rosenau charged that "in practically all other governments . . . in different parts of the world," research was "an understood function of government," and he urged that the United States, through the Public Health Service, be allowed to expand in this direction as well.[34]

California Representative Clarence F. Lea queried Rosenau about nongovernmental research activities and asked if research could be organized in such a manner as to yield a profit to those who engaged in it. Rosenau replied, "The greatest reward I know of in scientific work of this kind is the sole satisfaction which one has. There is no financial reward that comes or is expected by those who devote themselves to this particular kind of work."[35] The federal government, Rosenau contended, could best assist research by "coordinating, stimulating, advising, and cooperating"—all things that an expansion of the research capabilities of the Hygienic Laboratory would foster. "No other agency," he insisted, "could tie all the loose ends together."[36]

Witnesses at the hearing also buried the old hatchet of states' versus federal rights in health matters. S. W. Welch and Arthur T. Mc-Cormack, state health health officers from Alabama and Kentucky, reported that there was only goodwill between their offices and the Public Health Service. Welch observed: "The work must be done by the states, the National Government cooperating. . . . It is not the function of the Federal Government to do public health work in Alabama. It is the function of the Federal Government to come to Alabama and teach me how to do public health work in Alabama."[37]

Other speakers noted inequities between medical and other personnel in the Service. George W. Fuller, representing the American Society of Civil Engineers and the American Public Health Association (APHA), pointed out, for example, that nonmedical Service employees had to pay transportation expenses for their dependents whenever they were reassigned. This was not the case with regular medical officers.[38] He commented further that this situation "tended to discourage, in fact . . . almost prevent, the entrance of new men into the service."

S. W. Welch and Milton Rosenau joined Fuller in advocating commissions for nonmedical personnel. Welch focused on the inequitable disability compensation between members of the Commissioned Corps and civil servants. "If an engineer goes out with a surgeon to investigate a disease," he said, "if the surgeon is infected and goes down with the disease for a period of two years, he gets three-fourths pay during that time. If the engineer goes down, he gets $60 a month. Well, he has exposed his life just as much as the doctor has, and is entitled to the same protection from the Federal Government."[39] Rosenau spoke about what he felt was a "misconception" of certain congressmen as to the quasi-military organization of the Service. He likened the commissions of the Service to those of "a judge, or a consul, or a collector of customs, or a postmaster at one of the large stations."[40] The uniform, Rosenau continued, was worn "only occasionally; for example, when one is on inspection duty." It was a "sort of badge of office" and was "simply helpful in the work required of Service officers." The Service had "no military organization," he stressed, "nor is it military in spirit nor should it be nor will it ever be."

Although the overall tenor of the hearings on the Parker bill was favorable, the Sixty-Ninth Congress adjourned without taking action on it. The spring of 1927 was spent by proponents of both the Ransdell and Parker bills in seeking additional endorsements for the measures. Former Surgeon General Rupert Blue obtained support from the United

States Chamber of Commerce for the Parker bill. In a letter to Blue thanking him for his efforts, Surgeon General Cumming expressed his lack of enthusiasm for the sinking ship that was the national health movement–backed section one of the bill—the provision to transfer agencies into the Public Health Service. *"Entre nous,"* he said, "I shall not grieve very much if paragraph one is changed."[41]

Charles Holmes Herty, meanwhile, was soliciting endorsements for Ransdell's Senate bill that combined the National Institute of Health proposal with the provisions of the Parker bill. He obtained in April a resolution in support of S. 5835 from the American Chemical Society. His next goal was endorsement by the American Medical Association. In early May Herty wrote to Acting Surgeon General C. C. Pierce, soliciting his help.[42] Pierce replied to Herty's letter, pointing out that the AMA had already endorsed the original Parker bill. "Senator Ransdell's bill now includes all the provision of the Parker bill," Pierce wrote, "so in passing this resolution the American Medical Association has already approved the principles embodied in S. 5835. I do not know whether it would be wise to bring up the subject at this meeting of the American Medical Association."[43] Herty quickly replied to Pierce, stressing that it was indeed necessary to get a new endorsement because "the primary interest of the Chemical Foundation is in the provisions for greater opportunities for fundamental research by the Public Health Service, and we believe that this carries a public appeal which will hasten the enactment of this legislation."[44] The endorsement was ultimately secured. Herty wired Ransdell in Louisiana: "Your bill was endorsed by American Medical Association. Hurrah, now we can work."[45]

There was little activity, however, throughout the summer and early fall of 1927 on either bill. In October the tempo picked up again. By the middle of that month Herty was expanding his web of endorsements. In a memorandum to Francis Garvan he noted that the American Public Health Association was meeting in Cincinnati; Ransdell had arranged for the Louisiana state health officer to attend the meeting and seek support.[46] Service leaders were likewise busy soliciting support for the Parker bill at the APHA meeting. Assistant Surgeon General Thomas Parran had replaced John Kerr temporarily as the officer in charge of the legislation, because Kerr was suffering from a debilitating illness.[47] Parran talked with many of the state health officers at the meeting, noting which congressmen each knew and could lobby.[48] James A. Tobey also attended the meeting. Parran and Tobey conferred, and Tobey agreed to "use his efforts . . . with the President of the Borden and Company to communicate with Mr. Parker and other members of the New York delegation."[49] Moreover,

Tobey suggested that a "concerted effort" be made to secure articles and editorials in "every major medical and public health journal" and in popular periodicals as well.

The American Public Health Association voted to endorse the combined Ransdell and Parker bills. Herty, never one to rest on any laurels, wrote to Ransdell October 28: "Now I am very anxious to obtain a similar endorsement from the American Federation of Labor, for I feel that labor has more at stake in this matter than any other group of our citizens. I am also going to try to get endorsement by the National Federation of Women's Clubs, for it would be a real tower of strength if we could get the women of the country alive to this subject and aggressively interested."[50]

In November the Southern Medical Association, meeting in convention at Memphis, Tennessee, endorsed the Ransdell bill. Later that month Herty received an inquiry for more information about the bill from his old friend Edward Marshall, whose 1919 interview had helped to launch the earlier chemo-medical research institute idea. Marshall commented: "It occurs to me that you fellows have got a fight on your hands which will be one of the wonders of the world. The Ransdell bill is an exceedingly fascinating idea."[51]

Encouraged by the spate of endorsements, Ransdell introduced S. 871 into the newly convened Seventieth Congress. The bill was identical to S. 5835, containing provisions of both the Ransdell and Parker proposals. Ransdell and Herty continued their efforts to line up support for the extension of biomedical research in the months before hearings on the bill were scheduled. In a speech to a joint meeting of the Virginia section of the American Chemical Society and the Women's Club of Virginia, Herty revealed his conversion to the belief that federal sponsorship of a research institute was completely acceptable. Speaking of the proposed National Institute of Health, he said:

> Fortunately it is not necessary to make a house-to-house campaign to solicit funds for such an undertaking. The machinery is already provided— appropriations by Congress from the Federal taxes. . . . Remembering that . . . [the problem of illness] is fundamentally chemical, it will doubtless amaze you to learn that of the many millions of public funds appropriated last year, only thirty to forty thousand dollars were available for the chemical research work of the hygienic laboratory of the United States Public Health Service.[52]

In taking his message to all who would listen, Herty went to Battle Creek Michigan to speak at the Third Race Betterment Conference. In a memorandum to Garvan he exulted: "I broke loose from the conventional style of presentation, and put the question right squarely up to the audience as to what they were doing to support fundamental research on problems of health, and then explained the Ransdell bill, and urged their assistance in every way possible."[53] At this conference Herty had an opportunity to meet with several people who could lend prestige to the cause. Irving Fisher, fallen champion of the Committee of One Hundred's department of health campaign, presided at the meeting. Alexis Carrel, a Nobel laureate from the Rockefeller Institute, "sat in the front row and took in every word" of Herty's speech. Herty lunched with William J. Mayo of the renowned Mayo Clinic. The prestigious surgeon offered "to write letters to ten or twelve senators" whom he was "confident" he could influence "and urge their support of the bill."[54]

As Herty diligently sought endorsements and prepared for hearings on the proposed National Institute of Health, proponents of the Parker bill discovered opposition to their reorganization ideas that had not appeared at the 1927 hearings. Groups skeptical about the changes that would be made if the bill passed had apparently hoped it would die with the end of the Sixty-Ninth Congress. On December 5, 1927, however, shortly after the Seventieth Congress convened, Parker reintroduced the identical bill as H.R. 5766. At a conference with Parker and Assistant Surgeon General Thomas Parran, Carl E. Mapes, chairman of the subcommittee considering the bill, pointed out two sources of potential opposition. Government bureaus that might be transferred into the Public Health Service under section one of the Parker bill were already objecting, Mapes said. Moreover, he went on, there was objection "on the part of Congress to delegating such broad [transfer] authority to the President." Parran suggested that section one be modified to stipulate that agencies must approve their transfer before it would become effective. He also pointed out to Mapes that the president already had broad authority to transfer agencies into the Commerce Department, a clear precedent for the provision. Mapes did not argue. He did observe, however, that if the Service "wanted speedy action on, and passage of the bill," section one should be eliminated.[55]

Pressures against the bill intensified shortly after the New Year. On Monday, January 5, Parran reported that Mapes had made a formal inquiry "as to the possible attitude of Secretary Hoover concerning the transfer of the Division of Vital Statistics" out of the Commerce Department.[56] Four days later, following a strategy conference of top Service leaders, Parran visited Mapes at his office, "just prior to the Executive Meeting of the Sub-committee at 2:30 p.m."[57] Armed with relevant laws pertaining to the bill, Parran was asked to wait in Mapes's office while the subcommittee met, in case they needed to consult him. He was informed at the conclusion of the meeting that the subcommittee had eliminated section one entirely and reworded section two to allow the detailing of officers to other bureaus only when so requested by the bureau to which they would be sent.

In one swift action, the subcommittee had excised the heart of the original national health movement proposal for consolidation of government health agencies. What was left was wholly a Public Health Service administrative reform package. Once again the aspirations of those who wished to centralize government health activities had been denied. On this occasion, however, it was not the objections of the Public Health Service that had blocked the plan.

Mapes also told Parran that a representative of the dairy interests "wanted to be heard" on the bill and that "the committee was in receipt of a very extravagant letter from a man at the University of Maryland opposing the bill."[58] Because of this, Mapes said, the subcommittee had decided to give them a hearing two days hence "in order that it could not be said that the committee had 'shut out' any evidence."

The hearing on January 11 was significantly different in tone from the previous one. Most of the witnesses came to speak against the bill. The subcommittee's decision to delete section one and modify section two forestalled what would obviously have been vigorous opposition on these points. Several speakers, however, believed that the revisions to section two did not go far enough. They objected to the idea of detailed Public Health Service officers "supervising" the work of other departments. H. B. Thompson, representing the Proprietary Association, pounced on the word *supervise*. With support from representatives of the American Drug Manufacturers Association and the National Association of Retail Druggists, Thompson specifically opposed the detailing of a Service officer to the Bureau of Chemistry to supervise the enforcement of the Pure Food and Drugs Act.[59]

Three representatives of dairy associations also raised objections to the bill. S. M. Shoemaker of the Dairy Federation, an organization of milk producers, believed that the Parker bill gave the Public Health Service "rather complete powers over the Department of Agriculture."[60] Particularly he objected to the Service's Standard Milk Ordinance specifying minimum butterfat content and maximum bacteria levels allowed in milk. Shoemaker charged that by issuing the ordinance, the Service "deliberately took the position of entire opposition to certified milk," milk that was not pasteurized but produced under carefully controlled standards.[61] The pasteurized versus certified milk debate was a particularly sensitive issue in 1928 because Hygienic Laboratory bacteriologist Alice Evans had traced the cause of undulant fever to unpasteurized milk, no matter how clean.[62] Her evidence had not inclined many milk producers to change their ways of production, however, and they fought Public Health Service regulation of their operations.

There was opposition also, as there had been at the department of health hearings in 1910, from groups opposed to any extension of the authority of orthodox medicine. In contrast to 1910, when there were large numbers of witnesses of this persuasion, in 1928 one lone opposing witness appeared and one other group sent an opposing letter. Harry B. Anderson, representative of the Citizens Medical Reference Bureau, whose slogan was "Against Compulsory Medicine or Surgery for Children or Adults," rambled through testimony that was generally opposed to allowing the Service to recommend treatments for the population.[63] Chairman Mapes reminded him that "this committee has got to get down to concrete matters . . . and we would like to know just what your specific objection is."[64] Anderson's only concrete recommendation was to prohibit the Public Health Service from publishing or broadcasting on the radio the results of research.[65] A letter from the American Medical Liberty League urging defeat of the bill raised the "medical trust" allegation against the American Medical Association and charged that the Service was "completely controlled" by the AMA.[66]

Not all witnesses were hostile. One speaker came not to criticize provisions of the bill but to broaden them. E. Fullerton Cook, a representative of the American Pharmaceutical Association, testified that pharmacists should be included in the group to which commissions should be extended under the bill.[67] He also wanted the word *pharmaceutical* inserted in several key phrases of the bill to demonstrate the equal rank that pharmacists, in his opinion, shared with dentists and scientists. The lobbying effort by pharmacists was not a last minute power play. At the time of the 1927 hearing, Surgeon General Cumming had received a telegram urgently requesting him to include pharmacists in the benefits of the bill.[68] Shortly before the 1928 hearing, moreover, Cook had discussed the matter with Cumming and won his approval.[69]

As a result of the hearing, the subcommittee made only two substantive changes in the bill. The word *supervise* was deleted from section two, so that Service officers would be detailed only "to cooperate" with other agencies when requested. Pharmacists were also written into the bill in a number of places. Other opposition, the subcommittee believed, "did not . . . go to the merits of the legislation" and was ignored.[70] It was "really surprising," Mapes remarked later, that there were "so few people who are dissatisfied with the work of the Service."[71]

Overall changes in the bill were sufficient for Congressman Parker to reintroduce it as H.R. 10126.[72] The favorable committee report that accompanied the bill emphasized the importance of the personnel provision of the bill. Public health work, the report said, "is, or should be, a career service. It has become quite as dependent on these other professions for its success as upon the medical profession."[73]

Because Service leaders were so preoccupied with the fortunes of the Parker bill in the House, Charles Holmes Herty began to believe that he and Ransdell might have been mistaken in joining the two bills in the Senate.[74] Ransdell did not at this time share Herty's concern, but the events of the following month changed his mind.

Throughout February Ransdell tried to get Surgeon General Cumming to solicit support for the Institute bill from Lee K. Frankel of the Metropolitan Life Insurance Company. Herty had previously visited Frankel, feeling that endorsement by life insurance companies "would provide one of the most effective means for stirring up national sentiment in behalf of the bill."[75] Frankel, closely tied to the Parker bill, declined to speak out "unless he had direct word from General Cumming."[76] On Valentine's day Ransdell wired Herty: "Just conferred with Cumming. . . . Says he has delayed visiting Frankel pending report on Parker bill which he expects very soon. I insisted upon his seeing Frankel promptly and he promises to do so very soon. Am worried about this delay."[77]

Cumming finally visited Frankel but reported to Herty that they both considered it ill advised for Frankel to come out in favor of the proposed institute and its $10 million appropriation at this time. Privately to Garvan, Herty expressed his disillusionment with Cumming. "Frankly I think we have been double-crossed somewhat," he wrote, "for when I telephoned Frankel . . . he had a very different recollection of the original conversation we had at luncheon at the Metropolitan Life, so I decided to lay off any accusations."[78]

Ransdell's pressure on the Service became the topic of a staff conference on February 18.[79] Cumming's version of his conversation with Ransdell bespoke surprise at the senator's lack of comprehension of the political liability the large appropriation for the proposed Institute carried. He reported that Ransdell had offered to separate his bill from the Parker bill in the Senate, if the provisions of the combined bill "would embarrass the Surgeon General." Cumming also related the discussion he had had with Lee K. Frankel about the Ransdell bill. Unbeknownst to Ransdell and Herty, the Ransdell bill had found a potential supporter in James A. Tobey. Present at the meeting with Frankel, Tobey had suggested that "the health agencies get behind the Ransdell bill and drop the Parker bill in its present form," since his prized section one had been eliminated. Frankel and Metropolitan Life president Haley Fiske had dismissed Tobey's idea, however. Cumming presented all of this information to his advisors, but they reached no decision "as to what steps were indicated in connection with the Ransdell bill."

Five days later another conference was held on the two bills.[80] Strategy with regard to the Parker bill was clear. Cumming, with the support of Commerce Secretary Herbert Hoover, who was "very favorable" to the Parker bill, would request Wesley Jones, chairman of the Senate Commerce Committee, to introduce the House version of the bill into the Senate. This move, it was hoped, would prevent the bill "from being sent to the Finance Committee of the Senate," a committee not likely to act favorably on it because of its chairman, Reed Smoot. The staff also noted with pleasure that Frederic A. Delano, philanthropist and cousin to Franklin D. Roosevelt, favored the Parker bill. Delano did not think, however, that "the Ransdell bill in its present form" was "practicable of passage at this time." Because he appreciated the interest of Senator Ransdell in public health, however, Delano had suggested that "if feasible some sections of the Ransdell bill be incorporated into the Parker bill so as not to offend the Senator." Obviously, the Ransdell bill was considered by the Service a somewhat embarrassing anomaly at this time.

Ransdell read the reaction of the Service correctly and moved to separate the two bills. On February 27 he introduced S. 3391 containing only the National Institute of Health proposal.[81] In this new bill a blanket appropriation of $10 million was designated "to carry out the provisions of this act." Moreover, the distinction between the Institute and the Hygienic Laboratory was becoming blurred. They were referred to separately in the bill, but the relation between them was not specified. Provisions for private contributions, fellowships, use of the facility by state and local health officers, and exemption of appointed scientists from the Civil Service classification act remained the same.

Not wishing to alienate the Public Health Service, Ransdell and Herty decided upon a new course. Ransdell determined to throw his weight behind the Parker bill as introduced by Senator Wesley L. Jones in the Senate. Once the bill passed both the House and the Senate, the way would be clear for Public Health Service support of the Ransdell measure. In the light of this strategy, Ransdell "thought it desirable to postpone the hearings" on his own bill for several weeks.[82]

On March 7 the Parker bill came up for consideration in the House of Representatives. Carl E. Mapes presented an overview of the subcommittee's report and fielded questions about the bill. Mapes noted that one member of the Committee on Interstate and Foreign Commerce had voted against the bill.[83] The lone dissenter was Alabama's George Huddleston, who rose in vigorous opposition to the bill. Huddleston acknowledged that he opposed the measure out of his "natural conservatism and hidebound distrust of new things."[84] His fundamental argument was not against the Public Health Service particularly, but to the growth of any agency of the government. "Bureaus," he said, "never consent to reduce their powers and never to reduce their prerogatives or their emoluments. They always work only one way, like a ratchet, toward more dignity, more stability, more power, and more pay."[85] It was not the teachings of orthodox medicine he opposed, Huddleston continued. He observed, however, that if "there is one thing that the modern world has gone crazy about, it is medicine, and in particular the immunization of human beings."[86]

Clarence Lea of California took offense at Huddleston's ridicule of medical advances. "So for as I am concerned," Lea opined, "the money of the United States Treasury will be devoted to no purpose that I approve more heartily than that of investigation and research for the purpose of discovering better methods of treating, alleviating, and terminating the diseases that come from germs."[87]

As the vote on the bill neared, a congressman from New York who had introduced his own bill to provide for mental health with an appropriation exceeding $5 million offered an amendment to the Parker bill for the purpose of making a speech about mental health.[88] His oration given, he withdrew the amendment. Mapes moved that the vote be taken, and the Parker bill passed the House without a recorded vote.

With this hurdle cleared, Herty and Ransdell hoped the bill would swiftly pass in the Senate so that Public Health Service officials would be able to lend assistance to the Ransdell bill. Herty wrote Cumming a note of congratulations; Cumming replied and said, "I am sure that you and Senator Ransdell will both do everything possible to assist [the Parker bill's] passage in the Senate, when we may, as you say, all join hands in an effort to secure provision for fundamental research.[89]

Unfortunately, the Parker bill did not fare well in the Senate. Senator Reed Smoot contended that the measure gave "the same status to the Public Health Service as that enjoyed by the Army and Navy, not only to the doctors, but to the dieticians, nurses, etc."[90] On March 27, when Ransdell was absent from the Senate, Smoot moved to have the measure "taken from the Commerce Committee and sent to his own Committee on Finance."[91]

Because of this turn of events, Ransdell decided not to wait for final passage of the Parker bill before proceeding with hearings on his own legislation. Herty proposed the week of April 23 but stressed the necessity of "getting a clear understanding with the Public Health Service people. I am afraid," he said, "their present unsympathetic attitude may lead to a very awkward situation."[92] Cumming, however, did not object to the hearings, and he agreed that Public Health Service officials would testify.

The hearing convened at eleven o'clock Tuesday, April 24. In addition to his expert witnesses, Ransdell had amassed an impressive group of letters of endorsement from distinguished health authorities. He read into the record communications from William J. Mayo of the Mayo Clinic; W. W. Keen, former president of the American Medical Association; George E. Vincent, president of the Rockefeller Foundation; Ludvig Hektoen, chairman of the medical section of the National Research Council; Louis I. Dublin, statistician for the Metropolitan Life Insurance Company; Frederick L. Hoffman, statistician for the Prudential Life Insurance Company; C.-E.A. Winslow, former president of the American Public Health Association; Milton J. Rosenau, former director of the Hygienic Laboratory; Ray Lyman Wilbur, president of Stanford University; William H. Howell of the Johns Hopkins University; Haven Emerson of Columbia University; and other less well-known public health leaders.[93]

The need for such an expensive federally supported research institute, the efficacy of accepting private donations, and the relatively high compensation of scientists at the proposed facility were the main topics discussed at the hearing. Several witnesses testified to the need for the institute. Reid Hunt, member of the American Chemical Society Committee on an Institute for Chemo-Medical Research and former director of the Division of Pharmacology in the Hygienic Laboratory, catalogued the advances in medical research that had come from government-supported laboratories in foreign countries, particularly Germany.[94] He defended the $10 million appropriation included in the bill as essential if Americans were to catch up with German contributions. "It is perfectly safe to say," he commented, "that those German research institutes, founded from 20 to 40 years ago, could not possibly be duplicated and equipped in the United States for $10,000,000, or for a good deal more than that."[95]

Treat Johnson of Yale University, also a member of the ACS committee, stressed the need for cooperative research—big team science, as it were—as the rationale for expending a large amount on such an institute. "No single man today can cover any one field of science individually and make progress," he said.[96] Citing his own work on tuberculosis, Johnson outlined the cooperation obtained with some difficulty among Yale, the National Tuberculosis Association, the Rockefeller Institute, and several other universities and private institutions. "We have no machinery," he testified, "no organization under central control where the various efforts and activities can be brought together, and we can have a council around a table like this, and all these activities can be focused and direction given to the best efforts of the research."[97]

Representatives of private enterprise spoke of the limitations on the private sector's ability to conduct biomedical research. Perhaps the most interesting statement came in a letter from George E. Vincent, president of the Rockefeller Foundation. As head of the largest private philanthropic organization in the United States, Vincent could well have spoken in defense of purely private funds for research. Instead he stated: "While it is true that progress is being made in our knowledge of these diseases through investigation in university laboratories and clinics throughout the world, it would seem to be a duty of our Federal Government to take an appropriate and adequate part in this world-wide cooperative work. The Governments of England and Germany have set conspicuous examples of officially supported scientific inquiry."[98]

The secretary of the American Pharmaceutical Association, E. F. Kelly, testified that drug firms tried "to do research work as far as possible . . . but it is impossible for us to go beyond a certain point."[99] The peripatetic Arthur T. McCormack, state health officer of Kentucky who had also testified at the Parker bill hearings, was also on hand to reject the idea that universities and private institutes alone could support research adequately. Instead, he envisioned a partnership: "The application of the knowledge," he said, was the responsibility of "the great foundations and the great universities and the Government itself, above all the Government."[100]

To impress upon the subcommittee the kind of knowledge modern research techniques could produce, Ransdell had arranged with Simon Flexner and Alexis Carrel at the Rockefeller Institute for Medical Research for moving pictures of cellular activity to be shown. As he commented on the film, Institute representative A. H. Ebeling explained the techniques of tissue culture, the method by which the photographed cells had been grown.[101] Ransdell, perhaps anticipating the practical question that his colleagues might raise, asked Ebeling, "How do you apply that to the diseases of human beings?"[102] Ebeling's reply illustrated the intimate relationship between basic and applied research. He admitted that "the direct practical application of some of these things is more or less remote," but pointed out that "in this particular instance" there had indeed been an application of practical value. Speaking about the production of "vaccine virus" for smallpox vaccinations, he said:

> It was produced in calves, and we conducted some experiments, and we found that it was possible to cultivate the vaccine virus in a flask by the use of a common medium and tissue obtained from the chick embryo, and that after a period of about 12 days we had a sufficient amount of vaccine that could be used to inoculate 5,000 or 10,000 people. In other words, it is a huge step forward. The way has been opened up to the direct practical application of this method of tissue culture, which avoids the necessity of continued vaccination of animals to keep up the supply of vaccine virus.[103]

Assistant Surgeon General John Kerr spoke for the Public Health Service in relation to expanded research. Having been the director of the Scientific Research Division of the Service for a number of years, Kerr more than other Service officials seemed attuned to Ransdell's vision. "While we have a number of hospitals for the treatment of beneficiaries," Kerr said, "our great field is the development of facts through research that will be helpful and effective in the prevention of disease. That is the natural growth of the public health work in the Federal Government."[104] Foreseeing the political difficulties in creating such a large institution, Kerr placed the responsibility of such a momentous decision on Congress. "I think the great need," he testified, "is for the representatives of the public to accept the principle that there is a great field to be filled, and that it needs to be adequately supported."[105]

The bill's provision to accept outside donations for the funding of fellowships had been modeled after legislation governing the Smithsonian Institution and the Library of Congress, both of which were allowed to accept private bequests. This section, however, raised two questions: Would anyone contribute? If so, would there be strings attached? Maine senator Arthur R. Gould put the first question to Reid Hunt. The Harvard pharmacologist responded that

> of course nobody can tell, but I do know that there are men with not enough money to found a Rockefeller Institute, for example, who are giving a great deal of money to universities. . . . I think it is almost certain that gifts would come. I can speak as an outsider. The Hygienic Laboratory here has the reputation of being an extraordinarily successful and useful institution, etc., that money goes much further in the Hygienic Laboratory than almost any other place in the country when it comes to research in these subjects.[106]

John Kerr dealt with the question of what strings might be attached to the donated monies. "I realize," he commented, "that any authorization of that kind would have to be surrounded with safeguards." He stipulated that donations would necessarily be "unconditional" and used only for "fundamental lines of investigation, and not to particular appliances and particular problems that might have a selfish background."[107]

Kerr also addressed the nature of the research that might be conducted and, as a corollary, the types of personnel needed to perform the work. He acknowledged that the Public Health Service already had broad authority to investigate the diseases of man and that the emphasis of the bill on fundamental problems, in his opinion, was in no way limiting. "[We are] now realizing," he stated, "that fundamental problems throw light on concrete problems." He continued his testimony, stating: "Heretofore the public and the governmental establishments have looked to the medical profession largely for advances in medical science and public health. I think in the future we may look to the physicists and chemists and other scientists to bring out new facts which will be the keystones to tie together perhaps existing knowledge and enable us to solve problems that we have been unable to solve in the past."[108]

Pursuing the question of personnel further, Kerr noted that "one of the greatest problems in the conduct of research is the securing and keeping of scientific workers." It was not only because of small salaries that this was difficult, he stated, but because of the type of research workers needed. He explained: "We have the need of men along narrow but very essential fields, that were we to discontinue would have great difficulty in securing positions. In other words, the work is not developed in other parts of the country, and there is no call for that kind of service."[109] Ransdell sought to broaden the discussion to the international exchange of scientific workers. "What provisions have we now in the law for taking our knowledge to these foreign countries, and sending our scientists over to those countries to cooperate with them or to bring them to us?" Ransdell asked. Kerr replied that the international sanitary treaty provided for international exchanges. "We have no funds, of course," he remarked, but "we occasionally extend the facilities of the hygienic laboratory to scientists who come and stay for a little time. Of course, that is a courtesy, without expense."[110]

Throughout the hearings, Kentucky senator Frederic M. Sackett expressed reservations about the omission of definite provisions for the organization and financing of the proposed Institute. When he asked Herty if he had "a definite scheme as to what would be the running expenses of the institution," how many fellows would be appointed, and "what it would probably require in the way of annual appropriations," Sackett wanted the kinds of details that Herty and Ransdell hoped to avoid. In spite of the fact that Herty's committee in 1919 had estimated annual operating expenses of their proposed chemomedical research institute at four hundred and twenty thousand dollars, Herty replied, "Those details have not really been developed as yet. It will depend upon the question, first, whether Congress is disposed to develop a matter of this kind."[111] Ransdell added that his intention was to give the enterprise "a good start, feeling that if Congress ever established such an institution as this, money would be appropriated thereafter to carry it forward."[112]

Ransdell realized that the bill as written would not easily pass the subcommittee. He summarized the problems and potential solutions in a letter to Herty:

> My plan is to convene my sub-committee very soon and make a report to the full commerce committee in the hope of favorable action from it. In this connection Senator Sackett suggested to me that we change the name of the Hygienic Laboratory to *National Institute of Health* and increase its functions. . . . Both Senators Sackett and Gould indicated by their questions that the business details of the bill should be clarified. Senator Copeland will stand by whatever we wish, but it is quite important to have support of the other two senators in order to pass the bill at this session. I dislike to yield but it seems to me we can satisfy these two strong men (who in my opinion are real friends of the bill) by making some concession and at the same time retain what we most desire—a National Institute of Health—reasonable provision for a system of fellowships from the federal government—authorization to accept private donations—and general recognition of the necessity for much greater federal research of problems affecting human health, etc., etc.[113]

As Ransdell projected, the subcommittee recommended two major changes in the bill. The name of the Hygienic Laboratory was to be changed to the National Institute of Health and the concept of a separate institution abandoned. Appropriations were scaled down to $5 million.[114] Since the Hygienic Laboratory and the National Institute of Health were to be identical, the wording of the mission of the Institute was also slightly revised. The original emphasis on fundamental or basic research was removed from section one and the phrase "scientific research in the problems of the diseases of man" substituted. The stipulation that fellowship recipients should investigate "fundamental" problems remained.

When Ransdell submitted the revised draft of the bill to the full

Commerce Committee, he won approval with one further change. The sum $5 million was omitted and the clause rewritten to read: "There is hereby authorized to be appropriated out of money in the Treasury not otherwise appropriated, such sums as may be adequate to carry out the provisions of this act." On May 21, 1928, a new bill incorporating these changes, S. 4518, was reported favorably out of committee.[115]

This action, however, came toward the end of the congressional session, and Ransdell held little hope that the measure would pass the Senate before it adjourned. A filibuster over legislation to create Boulder Dam tied up the Senate, and the summer's political conventions turned the senators' thoughts from routine work and made them anxious for an early adjournment. Herty held on to a slim hope. On May 29 he wrote to Mildred E. Reeves in the Speaker's rooms of the House of Representatives:

> The filibuster in the Senate seemed to have proved the death knell of my hopes, nevertheless . . . there is the bare possibility that the bill may be reached before adjournment at 5:30 this afternoon. This is a slender thread to hold on by but until it breaks I am holding on. . . . I suppose it is my old habit of going to baseball games and never giving up hope for a successful outcome, no matter how bad the score may look, until the last man is out in the last inning.[116]

The bill did come up that afternoon, but Utah's junior senator, William H. King, objected. "Mr. President," he said, speaking to the presiding officer of the Senate, "this is a very important measure as the Senator had said, and it would be the basis of the establishment of another department and call for an enormous appropriation in the future. I think, before we embark upon this policy, we had better consider it." Ransdell conferred with King and finally convinced him to allow the bill to be considered. Utah's senior senator, Reed Smoot, rose at that point to state, "If the junior Senator from Utah withdraws his objection, the senior Senator will object." Faced with this solid opposition, the bill was passed over.[117]

Shortly after Congress adjourned, Herty wrote to Ransdell and analyzed the objections of the senators from Utah. He speculated that Smoot's objection related to the provision of the bill exempting scientists from the Classification Act of 1923, an act that Smoot had strongly supported as a Civil Service reform measure. Herty reiterated, however, that "for the purpose of securing the finest types of research men for the staff of the National Institute of Health, it would be very crippling if we had to limit the salaries to those prevailing in

usual government scientific offices."[118] Ransdell agreed with Herty's
assessment and said he was "inclined to fight to the bitter end" to
preserve this clause of the bill.[119]

Herty and Ransdell were not alone in battling the conservatism of
the senators from Utah. Public Health Service officials were having
their own troubles winning Smoot's and King's approval of the Parker
bill. On the same day Ransdell convened the hearings on his bill, the
Parker bill came up for consideration by the Senate. The Senate
version of the bill, which Smoot had diverted to his Finance Committee, was not the one considered. Service officials had negotiated with
Smoot since that move was made and had agreed to accept a series
of amendments Smoot had suggested to the House version of the
bill.[120] Smoot's changes were largely technical in nature. They placed
limitations on the total number of appointments that could be made in
each grade of officer in the Service, set a cap on the amount of disability
pay that could be offered, limited the number of nursing administrators
that could be appointed in the proposed nurse corps, restricted pharmacists from rising above the grade of Passed Assistant Surgeon,
restricted the Surgeon General to an eight-year tenure of office, and
required the president to select new Surgeons General from within
the Commissioned Officers Corps of the Service.

There was no debate on the bill. All of the amendments were agreed
upon without opposition, and the bill passed without a recorded vote.[121]
A conference committee was appointed to reconcile the differences
between the Senate and House versions of the bill, and all of Smoot's
amendments were accepted with one exception; the Conference Committee rejected the proposal to limit the president in selecting the
Surgeon General to members of the Commissioned Officers Corps of
the Service. "The conferees are of the opinion," they reported, "that
the President should not be confined to the service in making his
selection for this important position but should be permitted, in his
discretion, to select anyone specially qualified for the position."[122] The
committee also added a grandfather clause to the eight-year limitation
on the term of the Surgeon General that exempted the incumbent
Hugh Cumming from the rule.

The report of the conference committee was agreed to by both
houses of Congress May 10. Eight days later Calvin Coolidge vetoed
the Parker bill.

The president's rationale for the veto was that the section of the
bill commissioning nonmedical personnel was unconstitutional. Draf-
ters of the legislation had carefully stipulated that any candidate for a
commission would first have to pass an examination prepared by the
Service. Moreover, a board of Service officers would recommend the

grade at which any candidate would be commissioned. Coolidge believed that these provisions "attempted to vest" in the Service board "and in the Surgeon General participation in the executive function of appointment of officers of the United States, which function can be vested in and exercised only by the President, with the advice and consent of the Senate, the President alone, the courts of law, and heads of departments."[123]

In addition to his objections on constitutional grounds, Coolidge went on to comment:

> For some time past there has been a definite movement among various groups of Government professional and scientific employees toward militarization of their respective services, and I am impelled to oppose this movement from the standpoints of both economical administration and public policy. From an economic standpoint the method of appointment of the civilian personnel should be such that the force of Government employees can be increased or decreased as the needs of the service or condition of the Treasury makes necessary. But more important still, I do not believe that permanency of appointment of those engaged in the professional and scientific activities of the Government is necessary for progress or accomplishment in those activities or in keeping with public policy.[124]

Reaction to the veto in the Public Health Service was strong, primarily because Budget Director Lord was believed responsible for Coolidge's action. A Service memorandum recorded the dejection:

> Now, after weary months, when both Houses of Congress have considered, amended, and passed the legislation, it seems hardly an act of good faith on the part of General Lord at the last moment to seek to prevent its enactment into law. Indeed, such action by General Lord at this time would certainly admit of no satisfactory interpretation other than a desire on his part to prevent the development and promotion of public health, which in the judgment of all sanitarians, is one of the most important functions of any modern government.[125]

James A. Tobey, analyzing the veto of the bill he had helped to create, noted in his column for the *American Journal of Public Health* that Coolidge's constitutional objections to the bill were "pretty far fetched . . . inasmuch as the system approved by law in 1889," the method of appointing persons to the Commissioned Officers Corps, had never been held invalid and was "merely extended to cover additional personnel" by the Parker bill.[126] Coolidge's opposition, Tobey concluded, was the result of the "baneful influence of the Director of the Budget." And although Budget Director Lord and Senator Smoot "seem to be having the last laugh," he stated optimistically, "triumph for public health is only postponed, not prevented."[127]

The Coolidge administration had hampered the work of the Public Health Service, but proponents of the Ransdell and Parker bills should have taken heart that Congress held a more favorable opinion of federal health work. As representatives of the public, Congress reflected more clearly the positive attitude of the general population towards expansion of this type. The veto of the Parker bill was, as Tobey observed, a setback, not a defeat, and with the advent of a new administration the outlook for success became brighter.

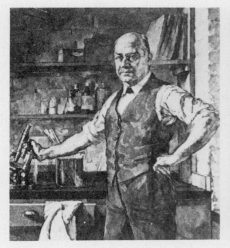

Joseph J. Kinyoun, 1887–1899

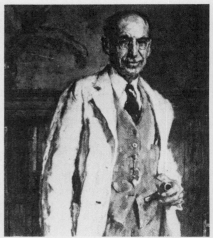

Milton J. Rosenau, 1899–1909

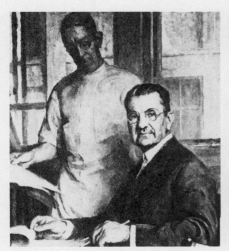

John F. Anderson, 1909–1915

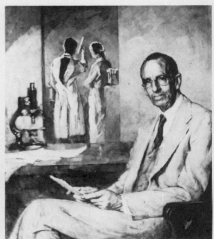

George W. McCoy, 1915–1937

Walmsley Lenhard's portraits of the directors of the Hygienic Laboratory and the National Institute of Health from 1887 to 1937 include details revealing their particular interests and areas of contribution. The dates are those of their directorships. These portraits hang in the administration building at the National Institutes of Health; photographs of the portraits courtesy of the National Library of Medicine.

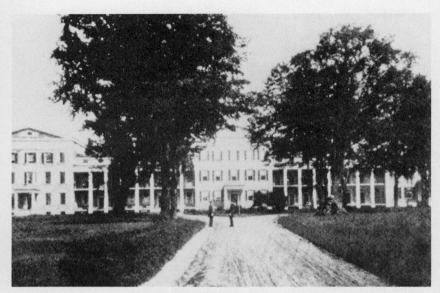

The Marine Hospital in Stapleton, Staten Island, New York, was the birthplace of the Hygienic Laboratory. The one-room laboratory's microscope and other scientific apparatus assisted Service officers charged with preventing the introduction of infectious diseases into the United States. Photograph from the Records of the Public Health Service, Record Group 90, National Archives.

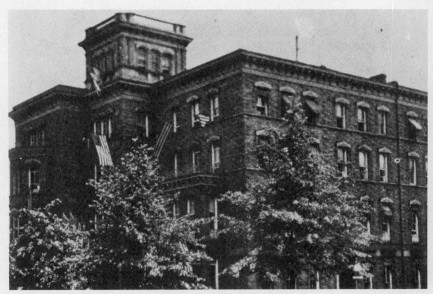

In 1891, only four years after its creation, the Hygienic Laboratory was moved to Washington, D.C. During the next fourteen years it was housed near the Capitol in the Butler Building, which was razed in 1929 for the construction of the Longworth House Office Building. Photograph courtesy of the National Library of Medicine.

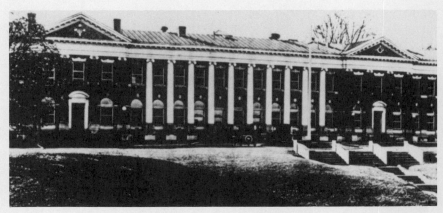

Congress officially recognized the work of the Hygienic Laboratory in 1901 and appropriated $35,000 for the construction of a building to house it. Erected in 1904 at Twenty-fifth and E Streets, Northwest, near the present site of the Kennedy Center, the original building shown in this photograph proved too small for the expanding laboratory. A south wing was therefore constructed, and, after the passage of the Ransdell Act in 1930, two additional buildings were added. The National Institute of Health occupied the complex until July 1938, when it moved to its present site in Bethesda, Maryland. Photograph courtesy of the National Library of Medicine.

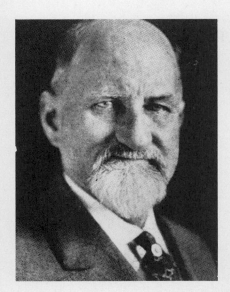

Architects of federal biomedical research policy in the 1920s.

Senator Joseph E. Ransdell of Louisiana sponsored the bill that transformed the Hygienic Laboratory into the National Institute of Health. Photograph courtesy of the National Library of Medicine.

Charles Holmes Herty, chemist and public advocate for increasing basic biomedical research in the federal government, sought popular support for Senator Ransdell's National Institute of Health proposal. Photograph from the Charles Holmes Herty Papers, Special Collections Department, Robert W. Woodruff Library, Emory University.

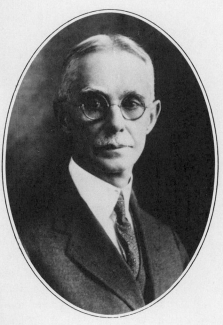

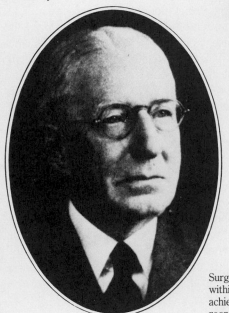

Surgeon General Hugh S. Cumming worked from within the Public Health Service bureaucracy to achieve passage of the Parker Act for Service reorganization and to enlarge the Service's research program. Photograph courtesy of the National Library of Medicine.

SEVEN

Perseverance, Compromise, and Success

> Some scientific discoveries and inventions have in the past been the
> result of genius struggling in poverty. But poverty does not clarify
> thought, nor furnish laboratory equipment. . . . The advance of
> science today is by the process of accretion. . . . A host of men, great
> equipment, long patient scientific experiment to build up the structure
> of knowledge, not stone by stone, but grain by grain,
> is now our only sure road of discovery and invention.
> *Herbert Hoover, 1926*

As the Seventieth Congress adjourned, the attention of legislators and the public was turned to the upcoming presidential campaign. Calvin Coolidge had announced his intention not to seek another term. The Republicans nominated popular Commerce Department Secretary Herbert Hoover, a mining engineer whose handling of the Belgian Relief Commission during World War I and the distribution of food after the war had won him admiration as the "Great Humanitarian." The Democrats organized behind New York Governor Alfred E. Smith. Prohibition, national prosperity, and the Catholicism of the Democratic nominee would be the key issues on which the election would turn. For proponents of the Ransdell and Parker bills, either candidate, if elected, would likely be more inclined to sympathize with their cause than had the taciturn Coolidge.

The American Public Health Association, which had promoted the Parker bill from its inception, attempted to keep the bill viable despite its veto by President Coolidge. At its annual meeting in October 1928, the association endorsed a resolution calling on Congress to pass the bill over Coolidge's veto.[1] This effort was in vain; no further congressional action was taken on the bill. The bill's proponents within the Public Health Service, moreover, seemed to have given up on Coolidge. Correspondence and memoranda on the bill were almost nonexistent from the time of the veto until after Herbert Hoover's inauguration.

Herty and Ransdell, however, continued their efforts to muster support for the National Institute of Health bill. Both believed that a strong endorsement by the major life insurance companies would be of great assistance. Herty, accordingly, talked with George T. White, chairman of the executive committee of the Association of Life Insurance Presidents, and with Lee K. Frankel of Metropolitan Life Insurance Company.[2] Neither cared to become involved with the Ransdell bill. Such reluctance, especially from Frankel, annoyed Ransdell because, as Ransdell wrote Herty, "it was largely on [Frankel's] suggestion that we delayed our bill until the Parker bill had passed, and because of the delay we did not secure passage of the bill at this session."[3]

It is unclear why the insurance industry was so cool to the proposal for a National Institute of Health. Official insurance company histories rarely make reference to lobbying efforts conducted by the industry, and the correspondence between Metropolitan Life executives and members of the Public Health Service does not illuminate the situation. One possible reason is that they viewed the Ransdell bill as competition to their own efforts at federal health correlation. Another is that as hard-headed businessmen who generally supported the Coolidge economic program, insurance executives could not favor the expenditure of millions of tax dollars on medical research. Whatever their reasons, neither Herty nor Ransdell was able to win their active support.

One other large group from whom Herty sought support with mixed success was American women. Individual women were enthusiastic in their response to his message, but galvanizing women's organizations in behalf of the bill seemed an elusive quest. In March 1928 Herty wrote to cosmetics manufacturer Florence Fabre-Rajotte: "If only we could get the women of the country thoroughly aroused on this subject it would prove a tremendous factor in securing favorable consideration of this measure."[4]

In his efforts to win women's endorsement, moreover, Herty had spoken before the Louisiana Society, an organization headed by Mary Goldberger, wife of Joseph Goldgerger, the renowned Hygienic Laboratory physician who had determined the cause and treatment of pellagra. Herty gave this speech a few days before the Commerce subcommittee hearing on the Ransdell bill, and after the meeting he wrote to Mary Goldberger, asking that she enlist the aid of the General Federation of Women's Clubs. "It would be fine if a large number of prominent women would show their interest by being present at the Hearing next Tuesday," Herty said. "I think that their presence would carry as much weight with the committee as the formal testimony of those who testify at the Hearings."[5] Mary Goldberger was enthusiastic. She attempted to interest the legislative committee of the National League of Women Voters and the National Parent Teachers Organization.[6] Apparently her efforts were unsuccessful. Presumably no large contingent of women came to the hearings, for there was no mention of them. Herty later complained to Grace Crocker, president of Wellesley College, that one of the "strange things about this movement" was the "ease with which it is possible to get the men interested in it and the difficulty in getting an equal interest among women. I had thought it would be just the reverse."[7]

Women's associations had been active throughout the Progressive Era on behalf of legislation to advance public health. They were strong advocates of the 1906 Pure Food and Drugs Law, the eight-hour day for women, the federal Children's Bureau, the Sheppard-Towner Maternity and Infancy Act, and a variety of other welfare proposals.[8] The political programs of these organizations emphasized broad social goals, and it is possible that the creation of an institute for medical research was perceived to be less important than more wide-ranging public health programs such as the Sheppard-Towner Act. The renewal of the appropriation for this act was an issue concurrently before Congress.

During the summer political conventions of 1928, the Democratic party adopted a plank in its platform on the problems of health and research, pledging the party to "adequate financial support," in order "to do all things possible to stamp out communicable and contagious diseases and to ascertain preventive means and remedies for these diseases, such as cancer, infantile paralysis, and others which heretofore have largely defied the skill of physicians."[9] The Republicans, in contrast, "overlooked the matter" of health in constructing their platform.[10] Possibly this was because they were able to capitalize on the prosperity of the country. To Herty, ever watchful for a way to promote the Ransdell bill, this omission needed to be corrected. He wrote to his friend E. C. Franklin, former director of the Division of Chemistry in the Hygienic Laboratory and at that time on the chemistry faculty at Stanford University. Herty urged Franklin to discuss the matter with Stanford president Ray Lyman Wilbur. Wilbur could, Herty believed, prevail on his close friend Herbert Hoover, the Republican nominee, to speak out strongly in favor of support for health in his acceptance speech to the convention.[11] Franklin did his job, and Wilbur spoke to Hoover, but the Republican nominee still failed to make the hoped-for endorsement.

So far as the election was concerned, party platform planks had little relevance. Herbert Hoover simply overwhelmed Al Smith, riding to victory on the wave of prosperity. In spite of the "omission" in the party's platform, Hoover's election was good news to supporters of the Ransdell and Parker bills. The Great Humanitarian was much more favorably disposed toward scientific work in the government than had been his predecessor. As secretary of Commerce, Hoover had increased government participation in a variety of programs, including public health measures. In 1922 he had arranged a merger between the American Child Hygiene Association and the Child Health Organization of America. The new organization was called the American Child Health Association and was funded by another of his organizations, the American Relief Association Children's Fund. Hoover installed himself as president of this organization and imposed a program of priorities on its activities; it became a "collateral arm" of Hoover's Commerce Secretariat.[12] In 1923 Hoover reorganized the private Better Homes in America organization as a public service corporation. The activities of Better Homes, which occupied a similar collateral status with the Commerce Department, included educational information on proper ventilation and other health concerns within the household.[13]

Hoover personally took charge in 1927 of the Mississippi Flood Committee, formed to coordinate relief efforts in that disaster. He was also interested in the study on the Costs of Medical Care begun in 1927 and chaired by Ray Lyman Wilbur, who became the secretary of the Interior after Hoover's inauguration. Speaking about the process of scientific discovery in 1926, Hoover displayed understanding of the needs of the scientific community, especially those members of the community who advocated cooperative research. He stated: "Some scientific discoveries and inventions have in the past been the result of genius struggling in poverty. But poverty does not clarify thought, nor furnish laboratory equipment. . . . The advance of science today is by the process of accretion. . . . A host of men, great equipment, long patient scientific experiment to build up the structure of knowledge, not stone by stone, but grain by grain, is now our only sure road of discovery and invention."[14]

In his inaugural address, moreover, Hoover devoted a short statement to his philosophy of public health. He said:

> In public health the discoveries of science have opened a new era. Many sections of our country and many groups of our citizens suffer from diseases the eradication of which are mere matters of administration and moderate expenditure. Public health service should be as fully organized and as universally incorporated into our governmental system as is public education. The returns are a thousand fold in economic benefits, and infinitely more in reduction of human suffering and promotion of human happiness.[15]

Surgeon General Cumming was particularly glad to see Calvin Coolidge leave the presidency and Herbert Hoover assume the post. Writing after Hoover's inauguration, Cumming noted that "the atmosphere around the White House now is quite different from that during the

Coolidge administration, and President Hoover has demonstrated several times not only an interest but a very intelligent interest in the work of this Service."[16]

Coolidge, however, continued to hold office until March 1929, and Herty and Ransdell worked throughout the fall of 1928 to win the president's support for establishing a National Institute Health. In September Ransdell visited Coolidge personally with the intent of "persuading him to include [a] strong recommendation" for adoption of the Ransdell bill in his annual message to Congress.[17] Coolidge refused to commit himself to the bill "until he had studied it," but he asked Ransdell "to write him about the measure between the 10th and 15th of November," during which time he would be preparing his message.[18]

Later the same day, Ransdell had an interview with Treasury Secretary Andrew Mellon. The secretary told Ransdell that he would send the bill and hearings to E. R. Weidlein, director of the Mellon Institute, for evaluation.[19] Hoping for a favorable report from Weidlein, Herty visited him in October. Herty later wrote to Francis Garvan at the Chemical Foundation about the meeting: "I had a very fine conference with Dr. Weidlein . . . in Pittsburgh last Saturday. He was badly mixed up about certain features which would have led, I think, to a rather unfavorable report, but I cleared all these up with him completely, left him enthusiastically in favor of the Bill and he assured me he would write a very favorable report to Mr. Mellon. I think this means a great deal more than appears on the surface."[20]

While waiting for Mellon and Coolidge to make their decisions, Ransdell negotiated with the Public Health Service. High-ranking Service officials were still stinging from the veto of the Parker bill, so Ransdell prodded them gently. "I explained fully," he wrote to Herty, "how important their bureau would become if our bill is adopted, and how, as a logical sequence, the Parker bill would follow it. They seemed grateful and promised to assist."[21] Neither their gratitude nor assistance was obvious in other circles, however. In November 1928 Charles H. Fullaway in the Bureau of the Budget appended this terse note to an analysis for Budget Director Lord of the differences between the previous and current Ransdell bills: "Incidentally . . . Surgeon General expressed himself at the recent Treasury hearings . . . to the effect that he did not think much of the proposed legislation."[22]

Correspondence between Herty and Ransdell was sparse during the autumn of 1928. Herty was making plans to open offices as a private industrial consultant. He moved from the Chemical Foundation offices on Beaver Street in New York to his new office on Park Avenue.[23] He continued to advise the Chemical Foundation, however, and was active in disseminating its latest book, *Chemistry in Medicine*. Edited by Julius Stieglitz, a member of the National Academy of Sciences who was chairman of the Department of Chemistry at the University of Chicago and a member of the American Chemical Society Committee on an Institute for Chemo-Medical Research, the book chronicled the role of chemistry in the physician's armamentarium. Herty's preoccupation elicited a jibe from Ransdell: "I think you must have been associating with lawyers who do not answer letters, for I have had no replies to several of my recent letters."[24] In response, Herty explained his silence and pointed to the potential impact of the new book in promoting the Ransdell bill:

> I think this book is going to have a powerful influence as an educational factor in the campaign for your bill. . . . If we can get . . . [President Coolidge] to read the Forward to this book . . . I believe we could count confidently on his effective aid, for he lost a son, Calvin, Jr. through the same lack of advancement of medical knowledge that Mr. and Mrs. Garvan suffered with the death of little Patricia, to whom this book is dedicated. Life is not all a matter of economy; surely the heart can play its part.[25]

Within a month, Herty had arranged for the president to receive the book through the agency of a personal friend.[26]

In mid-November Ransdell wrote to Coolidge, reminding him of his promise to consider speaking about health research in his annual message to Congress. The message was scheduled for December 4, Herty's birthday, and both Herty and Ransdell were in high spirits at the possibility of a strong presidential statement. On the morning of the speech, Herty wrote Franklin Hobbs with obvious anticipation: "Today is my birthday, but I have thoughtfully in mind the example of Mrs. Al Smith who asked the Nation to give her a birthday present on Election Day. You know what she got. So I am not going to connect my birthday with the day the President delivers his message to Congress, but am simply going to hope that before this day ends Congress will get a strong recommendation on health research legislation."[27]

Doubtless Herty felt a kinship with Mrs. Al Smith later that day. President Coolidge made no mention whatever of legislation for health research. Disappointed greatly, Herty and Ransdell continued to press Coolidge, despite Franklin Hobbs's conclusion that they would "have to wait for Mr. Hoover to push this legislation through."[28] One bright spot appeared during these frustrating days. Harvey W. Wiley, crusader for pure food and drugs, volunteered his support for the bill by writing an article for *Good Housekeeping Magazine* that presented the case for expanded governmental support for health research.[29]

With the coming of the New Year, external events combined with persistent seeking of support to yield positive results for the Ransdell bill. During the winter of 1928 and 1929, the United States suffered its worst influenza epidemic since the devastating pandemic of 1918. Influenza struck the Pacific coast in October. Reported cases peaked in December in the West, but the epidemic was moving eastward. The Northeast experienced the worst in late January and early February. Public Health Service surveys noted that 29.7 of each 100 people in cities across the country reported influenza, grippe, pneumonia, or colds.[30] The *New York Times* quoted Surgeon General Cumming as holding "little hope of any material progress toward the prevention of future epidemics until the influenza bacillus was isolated and a specific preventative developed."[31] Senator Royal S. Copeland, Ransdell's staunch supporter on the Commerce Committee and a homeopathic physician who had been health commissioner of New York City, did not miss the implications of Cumming's statement. "There can be no more striking example," he said,

> of the need for the enactment of your bill than the present situation regarding influenza. Considering the modern epidemics of this disease, we begin with the winter of '89 and '90. At that time we were absolutely ignorant of the causes of the disease and with no ideas whatever as to its control. In 1918 we felt the effect of the most terrific attack of modern times. We found ourselves without knowledge of the preventative agent. . . . Here we are at the end of ten years, having another epidemic, and to our amazement we find that no progress whatever has been made . . . since 1918, and practically no progress for a quarter of a century.[32]

The flu epidemic, if it did not actually convince key administration officials to back the bill, did not discourage their support. Early in January 1929 President Coolidge decided to support the Ransdell bill. The Public Health Service quickly followed his lead. Ransdell wrote Herty exultantly: "Just a few lines to tell you the leaven is working fine. Senator Sackett had a 45 minute interview with the president this morning and found him extremely favorable on our bill. . . . I have talked fully with Cumming, who is with us heart and soul, doing everything in his power."[33]

On this occasion Ransdell was correct. In contrast to his disparaging remarks in November, Cumming backed the bill sufficiently to have the Budget Bureau comment on his support.[34] Cumming also wrote Herty: "There is undoubtedly a growing interest in this measure. Now that the bill has been approved . . . I am taking every opportunity to favorably interest others in it."[35]

By the end of January, moreover, the persistent efforts to convince Secretary Mellon and the director of the Mellon Institute that the bill had merits reaped rewards. Mellon wrote a letter to the chairman of the Senate Commerce Committee supporting the bill and stating that it was not in conflict with the financial program of the president.[36] Both Herty and Ransdell believed their major stumbling blocks had been removed. "Certainly the iron is hot," Herty wrote Ransdell, "and it is getting time to strike, if you can only secure opportunity to bring the matter up for a vote."[37]

Ransdell attempted to do just that. On January 24, while suffering from a cold himself, he "made a vigorous effort . . . to have" the "health institute bill considered."[38] Delaware senator Thomas F. Bayard objected, however, despite Ransdell's vivid reminder of the "awful epidemic of influenza that is now sweeping over this country."[39] Bayard was "unwilling for the Federal Government to indulge in an absolutely unnecessary expense . . . when other institutions, not only in this country but throughout the world" were "carrying on the same work."[40] Ransdell, having lost this round, immediately wired Herty to help find "influential friends in Delaware and elsewhere" to appeal to Bayard.[41]

The following Sunday the *New York Times* ran a strong editorial in favor of the Ransdell bill.[42] Herty wrote comfortingly to Ransdell, "I regret to hear of your continued sickness. All the more reason for the quick passage of the Ransdell bill. You need *research*."[43]

Two weeks later Ransdell had recovered. On February 6 he addressed the Senate for more than two hours. With generous assistance from Senator Copeland, Ransdell again argued the case for the National Institute of Health.[44] Senators objecting to the bill argued primarily from positions of fiscal conservatism and states' rights, issues that had been previously discussed and were on this occasion quickly challenged by the array of facts Ransdell had amassed.[45] Senator C. C. Dill of Washington State, however, pursued a tougher line of questioning. "I want to know something about what the expense to the Government this institution eventually will be," he asked.[46] Since S. 4518 had been changed to read "sums adequate to carry out the provisions of this act," Ransdell could not provide an exact figure. To assuage Dill's concern, Ransdell spoke glowingly of the number of wealthy people expected to contribute to the Institute. Dill commented dryly, "If they do not, there is going to be a very heavy burden of expenses to the Government on the part of this institution." The omission of a stated appropriation was the bill's weakest point.

Although no vote was taken that day, Ransdell wrote to Herty that he was "watching like a hawk," and would do his "utmost to put this measure through the Senate before the close of the week."[47] He was not far off the mark. The vote did not come for three weeks, but the time was well used to solicit further support from the president and the media. On February 13 Herty "visited the editorial offices of the *New York Herald Tribune* . . . and urged them to give . . . a strong editorial" in support of the bill.[48] Armistead Holcombe, an editorial staff member of the *Tribune* and Kappa Alpha fraternity brother of Herty's, ran an editorial two days later that Herty felt would be "of educative value among those senators who have not time to read a more lengthy discussion of the bill."[49] The *New York Times* also published a pointed editorial in support of S. 4518. Noting that the bill was "not on the preferred calendar of the Senate" and could therefore "not come to a vote except by unanimous consent," the *Times* warned that "any Senator who would obstruct its consideration save for the most valid reasons, would be taking upon himself a responsibility measurable in terms of human life that might be saved by the service for which the bill provides or that might be lost because of another year's postponement."[50]

Ransdell again visited President Coolidge, who promised to do what he could, although he refused to send a special message to Congress.[51] Of more immediate value was the influence of the president's secretary, Everett Sanders, who appealed to Senator Smoot. The objecting senator promised to examine the bill, telling Sanders that "all he desired was to have a clear understanding of the bill before consenting to its being taken up."[52] Herty, moreover, pressed another friend, a distinguished New York City attorney, "to write a personal letter" to Smoot's junior colleague from Utah, Senator King.[53]

Although King had blocked consideration of the bill once again on February 21, he raised no objection when it came before the Senate Friday evening, March 1. Ransdell and Herty had drafted two amendments to the bill over lunch that day. The appropriations clause was reworded to read: "The Secretary of the Treasury is authorized and directed to submit to Congress not later than December 2, 1929, plans and estimates of appropriations necessary to carry out adequately the provisions of this act."[54] King "made it very clear" to Ransdell "that if the bill were so amended he would not oppose it." Writing to Herty, Ransdell commented that King "was on the spot" when he "asked unanimous consent" to consider the bill, and that King "certainly made no objection."[55] Senator Smoot, the other opponent of the bill, had been present in the Senate Friday morning, but he did not answer two roll calls in the hours before the vote was taken. Presumably he no longer felt strongly enough in opposition to the measure to be present. In very quick action the Senate agreed to the amendments and passed the Ransdell bill without a recorded vote.[56]

Two days later New York congressman William I. Sirovich moved to suspend the rules of the House of Representatives to pass the bill before Congress adjourned March 4. Supporters and opponents of the bill exchanged many sharp remarks. Michigan congressman Louis C. Cramton objected because "the proper committee—and it is a very able committee—has not seen fit for some reason to support the bill."[57] Although other arguments were also raised against the bill, peevishness at being what Cramton called a "rubber stamp" for Senate bills appeared to be the real problem in the House. Congressman James S. Parker, author of the vetoed Service reorganization legislation and chairman of the Interstate and Foreign Commerce Committee that had jurisdiction of the bill, stated that "the position of the committee . . . is not so much in opposition to the bill as in opposition to the method of procedure. We are not discussing the merits of this bill, because we know nothing about the bill itself. . . . I could not stand here on this floor and commend it."[58] Thus, although Sirovich argued that the bill was supported by the Public Health Service and Secretary Mellon and that President Coolidge had "signified his intention to sign it if passed," too few votes could be mustered to suspend the House rules, and the bill was passed over.[59]

Herty believed that the real reason for the opposition of Parker and Carl Mapes to the Ransdell bill, "which of course did not show up on the surface," was "a keen feeling of resentment on the part of Chairman Parker and Congressman Mapes against President Coolidge for his veto of the Parker bill."[60] He explained his reasoning in a letter to Franklin Hobbs:

> Six weeks before the close of the Session I discussed the whole question with Chairman Parker of the House Committee, and put the printed material in his hands, and [about two weeks] later I did the same with Congressman Mapes, during a fifteen minute conference with him in Mr. Longworth's office. But from the debate on the floor of the House one would judge that these two leaders were in absolute ignorance of the subject. This is a funny world. All of the House leaders with whom I talked had advised me to wait until after the bill had been passed by the Senate before pushing it in the House.[61]

Following this defeat, Herty and Ransdell commiserated with Public Health Service officials, who were still distressed over the veto of the Parker bill. All parties agreed that it would be advantageous "to have a measure prepared" which would "combine the features of the Ransdell bill and the Parker bill."[62] Surgeon General Cumming and his staff, moreover, suggested that "Mr. Mapes rather than Mr. Parker" was "the leading man on this subject in the House," and that adjusting the bill to overcome Mapes's objections would be wise.[63] Parker, however, was again designated to introduce the bill in the House. As a result of this planning conference, Ransdell felt confident that the Public Health Service would support the joint bill fully.[64]

Only one member of the Public Health Service staff still opposed the bill strongly at this time. Hygienic Laboratory Director George W. McCoy believed the bill was "fraught with disadvantages."[65] McCoy objected to changing the name of the Hygienic Laboratory because of "an element of sentiment" attached to the name as well as the "confusion in bibliography" that would result. He also feared that increasing the pay of scientists employed by the proposed institute would be deleterious to Service morale. Some of the "most desirable of the commissioned officers of the Service," he projected, might "resign their commissions and accept appointments in an institution which would enable them to spend their entire careers at the National Institute" rather than accepting the periodic duty station changes imposed on most Service officers.[66]

With most Service leaders behind them, however, Herty and Ransdell hoped for Senate passage of a combined bill during the summer's special session of Congress, followed by House passage in the December general session. Unfortunately, Parker balked at the idea of joining the two measures. Ransdell visited him in April and found him afraid of the section exempting scientists from the Classification Act of 1923.[67] Neither a letter from Herty nor a visit from Assistant Surgeon General Thomas Parran calmed Parker's fears. On May 4, Ransdell wrote Herty, "Am in somewhat of a quandary as to how to deal with Parker."[68] He determined to write Parker a letter that would require "a definite pro or con" from him.

While the issue of a joint Ransdell-Parker bill was pending, Ransdell made "a vigorous address of fourteen minutes on the radio over the N.B.C. hookup" in support of establishing a National Institute of Health.[69] He also paid a call on newly inaugurated President Hoover, which shortly yielded results.[70] On May 10 Ransdell received a letter from the new secretary of the Interior, Ray Lyman Wilbur, saying that President Hoover had taken up with him the "question of your bill" and had asked Wilbur "to be of assistance" if there was "any way" he could be "helpful."[71] Triumphantly, Ransdell wrote to Parker, asking for a definite decision on the joint bill and saying, "From what the President said to me in person, from the strong statement on health in his inaugural address, and from Mr. Wilbur's letter, I infer that he will assist us actively."[72]

Parker agreed to support the National Institute of Health bill, but he chose not to combine it with the Service reorganization bill. Ransdell, therefore, on May 20, 1929, introduced a separate National Institute of Health bill, S. 1171, and Parker introduced the identical bill into the House as H.R. 3143.[73] This version of the Ransdell bill spoke again of research into the "fundamental problems of the diseases of man," reinstating Herty's emphasis on basic research, at least in the section describing research to be conducted by Institute fellows. The new bill yielded somewhat, however, to those who opposed exempting scientists from regular Civil Service classification. Ransdell changed this section of the bill to read that scientists would be paid and classified "under regulations approved by the President." He also added a similar clause in section one, stipulating that the president should prescribe rules and regulations for governing the Institute. With these changes Ransdell sought to maintain a measure of independence for the type of scientists it was hoped the Institute could attract. On the question of appropriations, Ransdell rewrote the section once again. In this version, the secretary of the Treasury was charged with submitting to Congress "from time to time plans and appropriations necessary" for the operation of the institute.

S. 1171 was referred to the Committee on Commerce and sent to the Treasury Department for evaluation by the Bureau of the Budget. That bureau, however, was not pleased that the bill carried no definite appropriation. A memo prepared by Budget staff member Charles H. Fullaway stated that he was

> convinced that the proponents of the bill, notwithstanding the omission of an authorization for a specific amount to be appropriated, still have in mind that the Federal Government should expend not less than $10,000,000 in carrying out its provisions, in addition to the donations from private sources which the bill authorizes. It is apparent that the bill is sponsored by influential interests. The Secretary of the Treasury is in favor of it, and Mr. Mills [the Undersecretary of the Treasury] believes he can control within reasonable bounds the estimates that may arise should the bill be enacted into law. . . . The sole questions seem to be: 1) Is there a need for the United States entering into this work in the manner and to the extent contemplated, in view of the fact that it has heretofore been adequately sponsored and effectively carried on under private auspices. 2) Can we spare the funds, and would not a decision to approve the legislation open the door to the multitude of proposals of various kinds with which we have to deal.[74]

Treasury Undersecretary O. L. Mills took a stronger stand. He insisted that the bill should carry a definite sum to receive approval of his department. Secretary Mellon, furthermore, stood by his undersecretary. On July 25 Mellon wrote the chairman of the Committee on Commerce: "It is respectfully suggested that in lieu of the last sentence of section one . . . the following be inserted: 'There is hereby authorized to be appropriated the sum of $750,000 or so much thereof as may be necessary, for construction and equipment of additional buildings at the present Hygienic Laboratory of the Public Health Service.' "[75]

The sum suggested by Mellon was for construction and equipment only, but it was far different from the $5 million construction budget called for in the original 1926 version of the Ransdell bill. The new figure, however, was duly incorporated into S. 1171. Ransdell commented to Herty in August that the appropriation, in his opinion, was not a "very material matter. What we wish is to get the bill itself passed."[76] Ransdell's letter arrived while Herty was attending to a sad personal duty. Mrs. Herty died in August and was buried in Georgia.

Simultaneously with these events, a new Service reorganization bill had begun wending its way through the legislative maze. Parker's new bill, H.R. 3142, introduced the same day as Ransdell's latest Institute of Health proposal, contained revisions and additions designed to meet the objections stated by President Coolidge in his veto message.[77] The first three sections of the bill—authorizing the detailing of Service officers for duty in other federal bureaus, allowing Service personnel to conduct research at universities and private institutions, and identifying the Hygienic Laboratory as a field station of the Service— remained virtually the same.[78]

Major changes in the revised bill related to the personnel provisions that Coolidge found objectionable. Every vestige of what the president had identified as "unconstitutional language" was removed in the new bill.[79] Nonmedical officers were to be appointed according to "such regulations as the president may prescribe" rather than by a board of officers convened by the Surgeon General. This change was a fine point of wording, closely akin to splitting hairs, because in practice the method of selecting Commissioned Officers would remain unchanged. Similarly, the limitation on the length of the Surgeon General's term of office was removed since it was considered an unconstitutional limitation on the appointive powers of the President. In the section of the bill converting the Hygienic Laboratory Advisory Board into the National Advisory Health Council, it was stipulated that the secretary of the Treasury rather than the Surgeon General with the secretary's approval was authorized to appoint members.

Other changes in the personnel sections were more substantive. Scientists below the level of division director were deleted from the list of nonmedical personnel to be offered commissions, while dentists, sanitary engineers, and pharmacists remained. Presumably this was done because of Coolidge's specific objection to the commissioning of scientific personnel in his veto message. The provision that authorized commissions for the nonmedical division directors in the Hygienic Laboratory—the "Professors" of chemistry, pharmacology, and zoology—was left intact, however. The proposal for a nurse corps in the earlier bill was deleted in the new bill. A Service analysis of the new bill explained that this was done "in order to be taken care of more comprehensively in other legislation," but it may have been eliminated in order to avoid further charges that the Service was trying to "militarize."[80]

A new section was added specifying how officers found unfit for promotion for other than medical reasons would be separated from the Service. This allowed the Service to terminate inefficient officers instead of maintaining them at low-level positions indefinitely. Another addition provided for the appointment of an Assistant Surgeon General to head the new Narcotics Division of the Service, a division established in January 1929.[81] The earlier bill, moreover, had been amended to remove the limitation only on the number of senior surgeons that could be appointed. The new version reverted to the original 1926 bill in removing the restriction on the number of Assistant Surgeons General as well.

One major addition to the new bill corrected a serious problem facing Service personnel. According to a decision of the Comptroller General, personnel on duty in the field were entitled to treatment only at Marine Hospitals when they fell ill.[82] By 1929, thirty-two employees—including commissioned officers, laboratory attendants, a nurse, and a bacteriologist—had died from diseases they contracted in the line of duty.[83] Although many of these were stationed at Marine Hospitals, some were working in remote locations. The case of Thomas B. McClintic, who in 1912 contracted Rocky Mountain spotted fever in Hamilton, Montana, was the most notorious in Service annals. McClintic made the long trip back to Washington while gravely ill and died the day after he returned.[84] The new provision allowed the secretary of the Treasury to specify conditions under which these employees could be compensated for seeking hospital treatment at local facilities. Such a change was sorely needed.

The summer and fall of 1929 passed with little action on the Ransdell and Parker bills. Called into special session, Congress was preoccupied with debate on the Hawley-Smoot tariff, the highest ever in American history. The stock market continued to boom, and not even those investment advisors who counseled caution could foresee the coming Great Depression. Even after the collapse of Wall Street in October, the severity of the economic situation was apparently not yet evident.

No reference to the broader economic situation was introduced into the discussion of either bill.

Service memoranda on the progress of the Parker bill, which for previous versions had been detailed and meticulously filed, dropped off sharply during this period. Assistant Surgeons General John Kerr and Thomas Parran had been responsible for these records, and both suffered personal problems at this time. John Kerr, whose illness worsened, was detached from the administrative offices of the Service and sent to Hampton Roads, Virginia.[85] At the end of January 1929, Thomas Parran's wife died from cancer, so he was preoccupied with personal grief and with the care of his four small sons.[86] Because of this, Surgeon General Cumming took more of the responsibility for the passage of the bill directly upon himself.

At this time of increased responsibility, Cumming became embroiled in a controversy that threatened to affect the chances of the Parker bill in Congress. For some years Cumming had found the Children's Bureau to be a thorn in his flesh, especially after the Sheppard-Towner Maternity and Infancy Act was passed. A man of acknowledged conservative views, Cumming disliked the idea of social workers, such as Grace Abbott and Julia Lathrop, encroaching on what he believed was properly the concern of physicians. In December 1929 he wrote of his concern to the secretary of the Michigan State Medical Society: "It is time for representatives of the organized medical profession and the trained public health workers to get together with a common purpose of opposing such movements as are indicated by the Sheppard-Towner Act and similarly ill-advised ventures piloted by non-medical social workers."[87]

An extension of the appropriations for the Sheppard-Towner Act was before Congress at this time, and the proponents of the legislation had gained President Hoover's support. Cumming's outspoken opposition to the measure apparently engendered a warning of political reprisals from partisans of the bill. He noted threats that if he or the Service opposed the legislation, "there would be insuperable obstacles to the passage of the Parker bill."[88] Cumming was certainly not alone in his opposition. The American Medical Association staunchly opposed extension of the act. The acrimonious debate was settled by Congress in December 1929; the appropriation was allowed to lapse. The threatened reprisals against Cumming and the Parker bill apparently failed to materialize, because no further reference to the problem was made.

Continued difficulties with the Budget Bureau also delayed consideration of H.R. 3142. Herbert M. Lord retired as director of the Budget in 1929. The new director, J. Clawson Roop, was an unknown quantity to Service officials. Cumming feared that Roop might be under Lord's influence and might possibly refuse to approve the new bill. The Surgeon General, therefore, sought the assistance of William H. Welch, hoping that Welch, who had a "personal relationship" with President Hoover, would communicate with the president on behalf of the bill.[89]

Cumming's fears appear to have been well founded because initially Roop refused to approve the bill.[90] Shortly after the New Year, however, Cumming's efforts to reach President Hoover personally or through William H. Welch apparently succeeded. The Surgeon General wrote to a friend that he had gotten the bill "out of the Budget by appealing over their heads to the President."[91] In early January 1930, Roop approved the legislation with a reduction, from 110 to 55, in the number of nonmedical personnel designated to receive commissions.[92] The Committee on Interstate and Foreign Commerce so amended the bill and reported it out of committee without hearings as H.R. 8807 on January 28. The Senate Commerce Committee had likewise reported the amended bill on January 18 as S. 3167.[93]

While Cumming was preoccupied with the Parker bill, Ransdell and Herty were attempting to move the National Institute of Health bill through the Seventy-First Congress. Soon after the new Congress convened, Herty had written Parker, asking when the Committee of Interstate and Foreign Commerce would hold hearings on the House version of the Ransdell bill.[94] He received only a brief reply from the committee's clerk advising him that he would be notified. Again Herty wrote to Parker, prodding him for early hearings: "You will remember from the debate on the floor of the House . . . one of the obstacles to the passage of the measure was the inadequate time for committee hearings and report."[95] Parker replied personally this time, assuring Herty that he "had this bill in mind right along" and hoped that it would soon be brought before the committee.[96] Positive action on the bill came more quickly from the Senate. On January 18, Ransdell happily wrote Herty that he "was authorized to make a favorable report on our Health Institute bill by the Commerce Committee," and that he had presented the report to the Senate that morning.[97]

As both bills came ever closer to passage, the Citizen's Medical Reference Bureau—whose secretary, Harry B. Anderson, had testified against the Parker bill at the 1928 hearings—raised a strident voice in opposition. Mildred E. Reeves, secretary to House Speaker Nicholas Longworth, sent Herty a copy of a letter the Speaker had received from the group and clippings from the press setting forth their views.[98] Unlike members of the Committee of One Hundred, who had been stopped in their crusade twenty years earlier by such groups, Herty was not dismayed. His response reveals how far public opinion had shifted in the intervening years toward faith in orthodox medicine. "I do not think anybody could do anything with Mr. Anderson," Herty wrote to Reeves. "He is rabid on the subject, but fortunately I do not think he has any influence to amount to anything in his opposition to the Institute of Health Bill."[99]

The Senate remained locked in debate on the tariff until late March when the Hawley-Smoot bill finally passed. The two-month delay in having the bills come up for consideration began to wear on everyone. Surgeon General Cumming commented wryly to a friend about the Service's anxiety over the Parker bill: "I can't recall which guy it was who said, 'Hope deferred maketh the heart sick,' whether it was your old friend Solomon or Shakespeare, but there is a world of truth in it and the postponement has rather gotten on our nerves."[100]

An additional factor that certainly wore on the nerves of the Service but that may have contributed to the eventual success of both the Ransdell and Parker bills was an outbreak of psittacosis, the so-called parrot fever, in January 1930. The virulent infection spread from parrots imported for Christmas gifts and caused the deaths of thirty-six people before the Service was called on to investigate it.[101] Shortly after Hygienic Laboratory personnel began investigating the disease, a laboratory assistant died from it, and both the officer in charge and visiting researcher Ludvig Hektoen fell gravely ill. Work on the disease was brought to a halt; the building was fumigated so thoroughly that it was said sparrows flying over the roof fell dead. The danger inherent in Public Health Service research was never so clearly demonstrated as in this dramatic crisis in the capital city. Commenting on the possible positive effects of the epidemic, Surgeon General Cumming wrote to Thomas Parran, "I can see the possibility of getting a suitable building . . . and possibly a separate building for working on the extremely dangerous virus diseases."[102]

The Parker bill finally came to the floor of the House March 26. Carl E. Mapes, rather than the bill's sponsor, managed the bill, speaking eloquently in support of the measure. Some questions were raised about the increased costs to the taxpayer the bill would carry, but the major opposition centered on the reciprocal research agreement between Service personnel and nongovernmental laboratories. Ohio congressman Robert Crosser objected vigorously to the phrase allowing officers to be detailed "for the dissemination of information relating to public health," arguing that this provision would allow the Service to staff the faculties of private universities at public expense.[103] California congressman Clarence Lea supported Crosser, adding that the offending phrase would also allow the Service to disseminate "propaganda" for a particular school of medicine.[104] Lea offered an amendment to delete the phrase, but after heated debate over whether the Service could be trusted—or if not, whether the Appropriations Committee could adequately stop any attempt to provide faculty members at taxpayer expense—the amendment was rejected, twenty members voting aye, thirty-five voting no.[105] Other facets of the bill caused only brief discussion, and it was quickly passed without a recorded vote.[106]

April Fool's Day 1930 turned out to be a day of rejoicing for proponents of the Ransdell and Parker bills. On that day both measures passed the Senate in rapid succession. Neither Ransdell nor Herty were present in Washington when the vote on the National Institute of Health bill occurred. Ransdell, facing a reelection campaign that fall against the charismatic Huey Long, was in Louisiana "looking after his 'political fences.' "[107] Herty was attending to business in Georgia. The bill passed without discussion or a recorded vote. Lee Wilson, Ransdell's secretary, and Lois Woodford, Herty's secretary, wired their employers the good news.[108]

Bringing the Parker bill to the floor of the Senate that day, however, had taken a bit of political maneuvering. Unlike the Ransdell bill, the Parker bill was not on the regular Senate calendar. Commerce Committee chairman Wesley Jones, sponsor of the Senate version of the bill, believed that it would pass without objection if he were able to be recognized by the presiding officer of the Senate, Vice-President Charles Curtis.[109] Lucy Cumming, wife of the Surgeon General, stepped in at this point to aid her husband's cause. Mrs. Cumming, a personal friend of the vice-president's sister, telephoned her friend and persuaded her to intercede with her brother. That evening Senator Jones was "promptly recognized."[110]

Jones asked to bypass the Senate version of the bill and have the approved House version considered. Hearing no objection to his request, Jones offered one amendment, a minor change requested by Senator Smoot and approved by Surgeon General Cumming.[111] Quickly, the amendment and then the entire bill was passed with no recorded vote. The following day the House concurred with the amended version of the Senate bill. President Hoover signed the Parker Act as Public Law 71-106 on April 9.[112]

Congratulations poured in. Haven Emerson, chairman of the National Health Council committee that helped to draft the bill, wrote to Cumming, as did representatives of the American Dental Association, the American Mission to Lepers, the Metropolitan Life Insurance Company, and many of Cumming's fellow officers in the Service.[113] Cumming wrote to Lee K. Frankel at Metropolitan Life, "I shall never forget the important part which you and Mr. Fiske took in initiating this legislation and urging its passage."[114] To former Surgeon General Rupert Blue, a relieved Cumming praised the bill and commented that most officers of the Service failed to appreciate the benefits it would provide for them.[115]

With the enactment of the Parker bill, the Service gave its full support to passage of the Ransdell bill. Herty, Ransdell, and Cumming began at once to prepare for the House consideration of the bill. Herty wrote Mildred E. Reeves to assess the leaning of Speaker Longworth. She affirmed the Speaker's "continued interest in the matter."[116] Ransdell informed Herty that the bill would be in charge of Carl E. Mapes's subcommittee and proposed that the necessary House hearings be limited to Herty, Cumming, and himself.[117] As the April 21 hearing approached, Herty moved to acquire media support for their cause. He contacted John H. Finley at the *New York Times*, who cooperatively wrote a strong editorial that appeared the morning of the hearing.[118]

No one appeared in opposition to the bill, and there was only one new witness, Joseph Colt Bloodgood of the Johns Hopkins University Medical School. Much of the testimony was characterized by emotional appeals for the great benefits to mankind that would accrue from enactment of the bill. Bloodgood termed the measure an "epoch-making bill . . . the greatest contribution to health that has ever been made in the world."[119] Ransdell contended that the bill was "fraught with more potentialities for the benefit of mankind—for humanity in general—than any measure ever presented to the American Congress during the life of our Republic."[120] Herty, likewise, made an impassioned speech. "I sat in the House of Representatives on Monday, March 2 last year," he said, "when an effort was made to suspend the rules and pass this bill . . . and when I heard Mr. Longworth announce that . . . the motion had failed, I had a sinking feeling in my heart that I could hear the death knell of a given certain number of people who were going to die as certainly as the world, because of the necessary delay of a year before this research work could be expanded."[121]

Members of the committee were not particularly swayed by all the hyperbole, but neither were they hostile to the bill. Connecticut congressman Schuyler Merritt reminded Herty that "we all have sinking feelings in our hearts when the bills we are interested in do not go through."[122] Merritt and his colleagues were especially interested in the cancer research work conducted by Bloodgood. Foreshadowing the enthusiastic support for the bill that created the National Cancer Institute in 1937, members of the committee eagerly queried Bloodgood about his work, even though, as Congressman Sam Rayburn of Texas noted, it was off the subject of the Ransdell bill.[123] Bloodgood obliged with information on cancer treatments, but he quickly related his work to the larger question at issue. "The practice of medicine, gentlemen," he told the committee, "leads to a good income, undoubtedly, but it does not lead to the control of disease. . . . The cure for diseases is found in research laboratories."[124]

Surgeon General Cumming and Assistant Surgeon General John Kerr gave strong support for the provisions of the bill creating fellowships and authorizing donations to the Institute.[125] Cumming asked for two minor amendments to the bill. He wanted conditional donations to the Institute allowed if approved by himself, by the secretary of the Treasury, and by the body newly created when the Parker bill passed, the National Advisory Health Council. He also suggested that the director of the Institute receive the pay and allowances of a Medical Director of the Public Health Service.[126] Both amendments were accepted and made a part of the House version of the bill.

After the hearings, the committee dragged its feet in considering the bill in executive session. Even though Ransdell knew the committee had several other important matters before it, he, like Surgeon General Cumming two months previously, began to find the delay causing a great deal of anxiety. He wrote to Andrew Mellon, asking that he "send a good, strong letter to Mr. Parker, urging the importance of immediate action on this bill, or, perhaps better," that Mellon "call him over the telephone and have a chat with him. Perhaps I am a little nervous," Ransdell continued, "but the measure is so important, and has been hanging fire for so long, that I dread further delay."[127]

When the committee finally considered the bill, it made four more changes. The opening sentence authorizing the creation of a National Institute of Health was struck out. The bill then read simply, "The Hygienic Laboratory of the Public Health Service shall hereafter be known as the National Institute of Health."[128] Ransdell's statement in section one concerning presidential rules and regulations for the Institute was deleted, although a similar phrase in section four was left intact. The committee stipulated that scientists receiving fellowships could not be commissioned officers of the Public Health Service. Finally, a phrase was added requiring fellowships to be funded and maintained only "from funds donated for that purpose." Ransdell looked over the amended bill and wired Herty: "House committee amended our bill in several particulars but after carefully analyzing same with Dr. Lewis R. Thompson [of the Public Health Service] believe the spirit and intention of the original measure are maintained hence I shall urge its prompt passage by House and concurrence of Senate in House amendments."[129]

On May 15 the bill was reported favorably with amendments out of committee, and four days later it was taken up out of order by the House on the suggestion of Congressman Parker. In a complete about-face from the previous year, Parker led a defense of the bill in the ensuing debate. Many technical questions were raised about the proposed seven-hundred-and-fifty-thousand-dollar expenditure for a new building. Michigan congressman Roy O. Woodruff suggested that the facility be built "outside the District of Columbia" so that "the necessary acreage" could be obtained for future expansion. [130] Parker defended plans to build the new facility on the grounds of the existing Hygienic Laboratory, saying that those buildings "would be turned over to the Naval Hospital" should the Institute ever relocate. [131] Another congressman asked if the bill did no more than rename the Hygienic Laboratory. Parker explained the other provisions of the bill and added, "There is something in a name. 'The National Institute of Health' is very much more of a name than the 'Hygienic Laboratory.' "[132] Some concern was expressed over whether the Institute would receive enough from donations to pursue the fellowship program planned. Liberal New York congressman Fiorello LaGuardia opined that if private donations to the Institute failed, surely "the United States Government is big enough and rich enough to provide." [133]

When all questions had been discussed, Congressman James O'-Conner rose to praise Ransdell, his fellow Louisianan. He proclaimed that "the passage of this bill . . . means more to our country and those Americans that must follow us than the granite and steel palaces of New York or the marble and gilded monuments of the National Capital. We have indeed done noble things today." [134] Following O'Conner's speech, the House passed the bill as amended with a two-thirds majority.

Two days later, on May 21, Ransdell moved that the amended bill receive Senate concurrence. It did, without opposition. [135] On May 26 President Hoover signed it as Public Law 71-251, with Ransdell, Herty, and Assistant Surgeon General John Kerr in attendance. [136]

On the day the bill won Senate concurrence, Ransdell rose to address that body. He stated:

It gives me great satisfaction to realize that I am the author of this bill, which I believe is fraught with incalculable good to humanity; it is my dream come true. . . . During the years of persistent effort following the first introduction of this measure July 1, 1926, many men of vision and love for their fellows have assisted materially in doing the educational work necessary for its proper understanding by Congress. It is impossible to name all of them, but I cannot refrain from mentioning President Hoover; ex-

President Coolidge; Mr. Andrew Mellon, Secretary of the Treasury; and Mr. Francis P. Garvan, president of the Chemical Foundation. These four great Americans saw with clear eyes the possibilities of the health institute for preventing or curing disease, with its awful suffering and colossal economic losses, not only to our country but to the whole world.[137]

EIGHT

A National Institute of Health

With the far larger resources that the National Health Institute will
ultimately command, it should be capable of doing great things.
New York Times editorial, 1930

The day after President Herbert Hoover signed the Ransdell
Act creating a National Institute of Health, Charles Holmes
Herty sent the good news to the members of the Committee
on an Institute for Chemo-Medical Research.[1] A year later
he submitted a final report to the president of the American Chemical
Society and requested that the committee be discharged.[2]

A National Institute of Health had become a reality, but its expansion
into a large-scale, well-financed facility lay nearly twenty years ahead.
"With the far larger resources that the National Health Institute will
ultimately command," the *New York Times* predicted in an editorial
on the bill's passage, "it should be capable of doing great things."[3] In
the years immediately following this prophecy, however, a combination
of circumstances thwarted rapid advance. Most significant were the
harsh economic constraints imposed by the Great Depression. Hard
times hurt chances for expanded appropriations, indeed, forced reductions in the research work in progress. The vagaries of politics
likewise put restraints upon expansion, as did the conservative philosophy of Public Health Service leaders who directed the Institute.

Senator Ransdell was defeated in his reelection bid in the fall of
1930 by Louisiana governor Huey Long. After more than thirty years
in Congress, the persistent senator could no longer promote in an
official capacity his ideas for expanded federal research. Before he left
the Senate, however, Ransdell took a number of opportunities to speak
about his dreams for the Institute. In February 1931, he delivered a
long address to the Senate recapitulating the ills of humanity expected
to be overcome at the facility.[4] The Chemical Foundation, whose
financial backing had supported the institute concept since 1919, paid

the cost of printing two hundred and twenty thousand copies of this address and circulated it widely.[5] Ransdell and his supporters also inserted into the *Congressional Record* many laudatory articles and letters about the Institute.[6] One, for example, expressed the high hopes of the *Washington Star* for the nation's new medical research institute. The newspaper hailed the Institute as "the beginning of a new chapter in the history of medicine; a new contribution by the United States to medical knowledge of the most far-reaching influence in the relief of human suffering."[7]

Within a month of the bill's enactment, moreover, Ransdell had been able to announce with pride the first large donation to the fellowship program of the Institute. The Chemical Foundation gave one hundred thousand dollars, the income from which was "to be used for one or more fellowships in basic chemical research in matters pertaining to the public health."[8] Ransdell wrote a gracious note to Francis Garvan, president of the Chemical Foundation, thanking him for the "princely donation" and expressing the hope that it was "the harbinger of many others in the near future."[9]

Unfortunately for Ransdell and the Institute, the Great Depression crushed the realization of this dream. The depth and severity of the economic collapse, however, were not at first apparent. Knowing he was leaving the Senate, Ransdell made plans to develop an unofficial, private organization to solicit funds for fellowships at the National Institute of Health. He had two motives for this undertaking. "The first," he said in a letter to President Hoover, "was the laudable ambition to have my health dream come true as far as any personal efforts could avail, and the second was the necessity of employment to earn a living after leaving Congress."[10]

In December 1930, Ransdell visited Hoover for help in locating "generous philanthropists" to underwrite the cost of the proposed organization, which was to be called the Conference Board of the National Institute of Health.[11] Ransdell sought $20,000 to $25,000 annually for the Conference Board's activities. Hoover offered to secure $10,000 per year for two years from his American Relief Association Children's Fund if Ransdell could find a matching amount from another source.[12] Once again the Chemical Foundation proved a stalwart supporter. Francis Garvan agreed to provide the additional $10,000 per year for the first two years of the Conference Board's existence.[13] Even with these firm financial commitments, the senator apparently met with some difficulty in acquiring prominent board members until Surgeon General Cumming came to his assistance.[14]

The organizational meeting of the Conference Board was held March 18, 1931, in Cumming's office.[15] The board of directors elected at that meeting were William H. Welch and Hugh H. Young of the Johns Hopkins Medical School, former president of the American Medical Association Frank Billings, philanthropist Frederic A. Delano, Francis Garvan of the Chemical Foundation, Charles Holmes Herty, and Ransdell as executive director.[16] The mission of the Conference Board approved by the new directors was "to assist, in an unofficial way, the Public Health Service in executing the Act which created the National Institute of Health, by making known to people who are interested in public health the aims and needs of the Institute through proper educational methods and otherwise."[17] The program for the Conference Board's first year, however, was to be entirely educational. "Owing to the business depression and the necessity for discreet advertising of the Institute," Executive Director Ransdell stated, "it was deemed best . . . not to seek contributions."[18]

From an office at the National Press Club, Ransdell plunged into his new job with the same fervor he had brought to legislative battles in the Senate. During the first year of its existence, the Conference Board, under Ransdell's direction, prepared "approximately 25 news articles concerning the history, work, and aims of the National Institute of Health," and convinced the editor of the *U.S. Daily* to deliver an address on the Institute "in his series of radio talks entitled 'Our Government.' "[19] Ransdell himself, moreover, spoke on the NBC network in March 1932 and in 1931 addressed the Washington, D.C. Parent-Teacher's Association.[20] During the next year Ransdell continued such activities and personally prepared two manuscripts for publication—a booklet to be entitled "A Fight for Your Health—The National Institute of Health" and an article "from a layman's point of view on cancer" in collaboration with Joseph Colt Bloodgood.[21] Neither was accepted for publication, however, "owing to the depression."[22]

Even though no funds were solicited for the Institute during the first year of the Conference Board's existence, a few small donations were received. Regrettably, these were the only funds ever brought in by the Board. The Depression's impact can clearly be seen in the paltry amounts, which are quickly listed:

C.P. Wilder, Worcester, Massachusetts	$1.00
Dr. Frank Appel, New York City	5.00
Herman Nichols	1.00
Senator Royal S. Copeland, New York	25.00
Bird S. Coler, New York City	10.00
Conference Board of the Institute	15.00[23]

In mid-1932 Ransdell did not expect fifty-seven dollars to be the grand total he would be able to raise in addition to the Chemical

Foundation's large donation. He prepared to seek funds from foundations and wealthy individuals, reporting that "a careful survey of their activities and past and prospective gifts is being made. As executive director," he continued, "it is my intention . . . to pursue a quiet, persistent policy of letter writing and personal visits, looking toward possible gifts."[24] A list of about three thousand names "of wealthy Americans" was compiled.[25] On May 18 Ransdell attended a meeting "of prominent insurance officials and others interested in conservation of health."[26] Representatives of the insurance companies "indicated their deep interest in health research, but said that the provisions of their legislative charters prevented them from spending money for that purpose."[27]

In September, after consultation with Assistant Surgeon General L. R. Thompson and with Carl Voegtlin, chief of the Division of Pharmacology at the Institute, Ransdell appealed to the Josiah Macy, Jr. Foundation "for assistance in carrying on cancer research at the Institute."[28] He proposed to relatives of the late Edith Rockefeller McCormick that "the creation of one or more fellowships in cancer research at the Institute would be a proper and fitting memorial to her," a victim of cancer.[29] Likewise, Ransdell approached Alice Roosevelt Longworth about establishing a fellowship "for the special studies of pneumonia," the disease that caused the death of her husband, Speaker Nicholas Longworth.[30] Reporting on these activities, Ransdell attempted to be optimistic in the face of oppressive economic reality. He said: "Financial difficulties, which all have encountered, prevented favorable replies to these appeals, but it is heartening to know that the persons and organizations approached on this matter spoke highly of the work of the Institute of Health, and attributed their failure to assist to the depleted condition of their treasuries."[31]

The two-year period for which Ransdell's financial backers had pledged their support of the Conference Board ended in March 1933—when the Depression reached its nadir. As Franklin Delano Roosevelt prepared to assume the presidency, one-third of the population of some states was jobless; the banking system had disintegrated; and total national income had dropped from over $80 billion to less than $50 billion.[32] Neither group that had supported the Conference Board was able to extend funds any longer.

Ransdell cast about for an alternative plan. William L. Dunne, an engineer associated with Cuban sugar interests, suggested to Ransdell the formation of a new organization under the auspices of the Conference Board that could be supported by small contributions from a large number of people.[33] The proposed organization, designated the National Health Foundation, would be more broadly conceived than the Conference Board. It would promote education in health matters, "foster philanthropy," and act as a "medium of exchange" to "promote cooperation in the practices of the medical and allied professions."[34] To finance the organization, it was proposed that the foundation publish a popular health magazine underwritten at first by insurance companies and eventually supported by subscriptions. Ransdell was advised by J. C. Funk, director of the Pennsylvania Bureau of Public Health Education: "An editorial policy which would involve legitimate and ethical propaganda in favor of health examinations, of insurance, and, of course, stressing preventive medicine, would offer the insurance companies a medium to circulate information to the public which should favorably reflect itself in their respective treasuries."[35]

Ransdell won support for this proposal from a number of prominent health leaders—or at least the right to list them as members of the board of trustees.[36] The magazine scheme never received a concrete commitment from any potential backer, however, and members of the board soon began to reconsider their support.[37]

The *coup de grace* was given to the foundation by Surgeon General Cumming, who opposed the plan outright. He told Ransdell that he felt there were too many similar organizations, that he was "strongly opposed to any new health organizations," and that he felt "some of the existing ones should go out of business."[38] Ransdell had heard reports, moreover, that Cumming had used even stronger language about the proposal earlier. Writing to a friend about a meeting with the Surgeon General, Ransdell said:

> I explained to the General how much hurt I was to learn that he had spoken in such an unfriendly way about the National Health Foundation and my efforts along health lines. . . . When I indicated that the statement in regard to the failure of the two individuals to continue financing the Conference Board of the National Institute of Health was because it did not make good, or words to that effect, he said he had not intended to imply such a thing, and that the inference must have been the work of someone "desiring to make trouble."[39]

Cumming's opposition, on whatever grounds, effectively ended what was beginning to appear primarily a means for Ransdell's continued employment in Washington.

Before it was apparent that his plan would collapse, Ransdell had filed papers of incorporation, had begun to use letterhead stationery, and had adopted a corporate motto unabashedly appropriated from the Smithsonian Institution—"For the Increase and Diffusion of Knowledge Pertaining to the Health of Mankind."[40] By July 1933, however, the last remaining Conference Board funds were exhausted with not a penny of new support in sight. The dejected former senator wrote to the foundation's board of trustees that he would "not attempt to formally dissolve the National Health Foundation," but would "allow it to remain in statu [*sic*] quo for the time being."[41]

Ransdell returned to his plantation in Louisiana after the demise of the Conference Board and the National Health Foundation. He lived quietly, out of politics, until his death at age ninety-six in 1954. Shortly after the Ransdell bill passed in 1930, the *Washington Star* had predicted that to Ransdell would go "first honors for this great humanitarian measure," and the Institute he had founded would be "a lasting memorial to his name."[42] This prophecy did not come to pass. By the time the expansion of which Ransdell had dreamed took place, most of the Public Health Service leaders with whom he had worked were either dead or retired. The interest of the new leaders was focused on the present and future, and Ransdell's name slipped into near oblivion.

There had been one memorial dinner in his honor on July 12, 1930, in New Orleans, at which Surgeon General Cumming, Joseph Colt Bloodgood, Charles Holmes Herty, and others testified to his contributions.[43] Perhaps Ransdell expected a building at the Institute to be named in his honor, but none was, and after his wife's death in 1935 he occasionally wrote to friends and Public Health Service officials, reminding them of his past achievements. Thomas Parran, who was Surgeon General in 1938 at the time Ransdell wrote, replied to one of these letters: "Dr. [Lewis R.] Thompson and I have frequently talked about you and the great service you rendered to the Public Health Service when you brought the National Institute of Health into being and aroused the interest of Congress in the research work of the Service."[44]

Parran went on to tell Ransdell of the expansion of research under President Franklin Roosevelt's New Deal policies, and although Parran commented that the officers of the Service were "forever deeply grateful to you for your foresight," Ransdell was not content. He later wrote to his nephew about his feelings of neglect and received a more sympathetic answer: "You are entirely correct in feeling that proper credit has never been given you for your work towards creating the National Institute of Health. . . . Your dream for the institution will probably materialize, though more slowly than you have hoped."[45]

As a politician out of office and a man lonely after his wife's death, Ransdell could dwell on such things. The man whose idea initially had inspired Ransdell's legislation—Charles Holmes Herty—was not so concerned with the allocation of credit. Having seen the National Institute of Health become a reality, Herty turned his energies after

1930 to the development of a system for making newsprint from southern pine, a process many had claimed to be impossible. Again, he was aided by Francis Garvan and the Chemical Foundation.[46] His labors brought him a variety of honors, including a Texas town named for him and the medal of the American Institute of Chemists "for noteworthy and outstanding service to the science of chemistry and the profession of chemist in America."[47] He died in 1938 following a heart attack.

Although the later mushrooming of biomedical research overshadowed the more modest expansion provided by the Ransdell and Parker Acts, Public Health Service leaders in 1930 were uplifted by the promise of orderly development contained in the measures. In April 1931, at the first meeting of the National Advisory Health Council—the body newly created by the Parker Act—Surgeon General Cumming lauded the previous year as "a rather remarkable year in the history of the Service—the most remarkable year since the creation of the Service."[48] On the council's agenda at that meeting was a discussion of many of the provisions of the two acts. Members considered the implications of their decisions carefully, knowing that they would be setting precedents in the interpretation of the legislation.

The Ransdell Act's provision for fellowships left a broad area for interpretation. Foremost was defining the kind of researcher to fill the existing position made possible by the Chemical Foundation's $100,000 gift. George W. McCoy, director of the Institute, pointed out the choices. "In a general way," he said, "we have two types—one to do work under fairly close supervision on problems chosen by the chief of the division—and the other type—which is what we have in mind for this particular position—is one quite capable of going entirely independently, working along some line closely related to the main field of public health."[49] After some discussion, Haven Emerson, William H. Welch, Milton J. Rosenau, and other distinguished council members advised that for the long term, assuming funds became available for many fellowships, the Surgeon General should be allowed "great elasticity" in selecting fellows to meet the needs of the Institute.[50]

The members' counsel was wise, but as a consequence of the Depression, no new fellows were appointed. The Chemical Foundation, in fact, was persuaded to allow the principal as well as the interest from its gift to be used in support of its fellow because of the low rate of return on investments in the 1930s.[51] Designated a "Research Associate," the fellow appointed was Clifford B. Purves, who engaged in productive research until 1936 on isolating and analyzing the activity of the enzyme invertase extracted from yeast.[52]

Another major consideration for the National Advisory Health Council was the provision of the Parker Act allowing the creation of new
divisions in the Institute. Discussion of this measure reflected the
broader areas of development emerging in the Service. Assistant Surgeon General L. R. Thompson reported that an internal Service board
had recommended the addition of divisions of physics and physiology.[53]
Council member Alfred Stengel of the Pennsylvania University Hospital in Philadelphia believed that the division of pharmacology "would
sufficiently take care of physiological developments," and he recommended expansion only "in the direction of physics."[54] Other ideas
were presented, including expansion into medical pathology, pathogenic microbiology, industrial hygiene, parasitology, and sanitary engineering.[55] Thompson pointed out that the Service already had in
Ohio what was "practically a sanitary engineering laboratory."[56] He
was referring to the Cincinnati water and sewage study project that
had been stimulated by the 1912 legislation allowing investigation of
water pollution. Council members finally agreed with the conclusions
of the internal Service board and voted to recommend the establishment of new divisions in physics and physiology.[57]

The Ohio water pollution laboratory was but one of three specialized
facilities throughout the country operated by the Service. The Rocky
Mountain Spotted Fever Laboratory was situated in Hamilton, Montana, and the Pacific Coast Plague Laboratory was located in San
Francisco. These laboratories had been developed to meet particular
problems; Assistant Surgeon General Thompson proposed that they
be made an integral part of the Service's overall plan for diversified
research.[58] After some discussion, the council accepted this proposal.

The role of the National Institute of Health in this larger plan was
also debated. Since the other Service laboratories focused on particular
disease problems, Thompson asked the members of the National Advisory Health Council whether they thought the Institute should be
"inclined towards purely basic scientific research."[59] A decision about
this was "very important for the trend of our work in the future," he
continued. The discussion of the council on this issue focused on the
difficulty in judging before the fact the applicability of basic research
to medicine. C.-E.A. Winslow noted the work of Mansfield Clark on
hydrogen ions and oxidation-reduction. "I think," he said, "that was
one of the most important contributions in public health made in the
last ten years in the United States. Yet it is in its essence one of the
most fundamental problems in chemistry."[60] An understanding of the
concentration of hydrogen ions and the ability to measure it accurately
was necessary to comprehend the chemical changes that occur in body
fluids, particularly blood, in illness. An understanding of oxidation-

reduction allowed explanation of a host of bodily processes such as the mechanism by which aerobic metabolism occurs in the cells.

Surgeon General Cumming agreed that it was necessary to support researchers whose work might not have immediate demonstrable value. Referring to the work of Claude Hudson, which later became "one of the most notable landmarks in carbohydrate chemistry," he said: "I do not know of any possible connection Professor Hudson's work on sugars will have to public health. Yet you never can tell."[61] Despite the strong conviction expressed that basic research was central to biomedical science, members of the council were reluctant to commit the National Institute of Health solely to fundamental studies. Milton J. Rosenau, the former director of the Hygienic Laboratory who had presided over its first period of expansion at the turn of the century, summed up the attitude of the council. "We all like to see a continuation of the advancement of the fundamental sciences but in no way should that discourage its practical applications to other work."[62]

This optimistic discussion and planning in April 1931 set the tone for future development at the National Institute of Health, but the recommendation for immediate expansion ran afoul of the economy. The proposed divisions of physics and physiology were not created because of severe budgetary restrictions in subsequent years. In 1933, for example, Surgeon General Cumming submitted a plan requested by the Bureau of the Budget to reduce Service expenditures for fiscal year 1934 by nearly 25 percent, including a $12,475 reduction in the planned $54,775 allotment for the activities of the National Institute of Health.[63] Cumming fought hard for the maintenance of salaries for his commissioned officers and for research work being pursued in the field at this time. One proposal from the Budget Office suggested the closing of the Rocky Mountain Spotted Fever Laboratory, which produced a vaccine used in preventing that disease. Cumming argued forcibly against this move. "If the government should discontinue this activity in the light of our present knowledge," he admonished the undersecretary of the Treasury in charge of the Budget, "the persons responsible for such action would in my opinion be morally responsible for the deaths which will occur as a result of the lack of this material."[64] His view prevailed; scarce though monies were in 1933, funds were allocated to continue the operation of the Hamilton laboratory.

Cumming was successful in efforts to prevent the dismantling of public health work during the Depression. He was not as adept in responding vigorously when President Roosevelt's New Deal policies opened the way to even more rapid expansion than that proposed in 1931. Roosevelt and his supporters were committed to the concept that government should play an active part in the social welfare of the nation. They also abjured the balanced budget in favor of stimulating the economy through deficit spending. Together, these two policies favored the rapid expansion of public health programs, including research. Cumming, who was basically a conservative leader, and George McCoy, director of the Institute who shared his views, were witnessing a major change in political philosophy that would ultimately generate the kind of large-scale research envisioned by Herty and Ransdell. Neither Cumming nor McCoy could conscientiously support the new plans. McCoy, in particular, believed that his carefully nurtured research organization was threatened.

Born in Pennsylvania of Scotch descent, McCoy took his M.D. in 1898 at the University of Pennsylvania Medical School.[65] After joining the Service in 1900, he worked with Surgeon General Rupert Blue on plague in California. In 1909 he was appointed director of the United States Plague Laboratory in San Francisco. During his work on plague, McCoy discovered the bacterium of tularemia. In 1911 he became director of the Service's Leprosy Investigation Station at Honolulu, and he rapidly became an authority on that disease. Appointed director of the Hygienic Laboratory in 1915, McCoy held the position until 1937. His Scotch ancestry, according to many who knew him, showed in his opposition to any trappings "such as expensive rugs, fine desks or paintings in his own or any other office."[66] He was almost universally respected as a scientist and as an administrator who allowed his staff the greatest latitude in pursuing their scientific interests.[67] McCoy apparently viewed his staff as family members; this personal concern, however, led him to oppose large-scale expansion that might threaten the intimate nature of the Laboratory.

McCoy had opposed the provisions of the Ransdell bill and was not convinced even after its enactment that its provisions were wise. He feared that the fellowship program, for example, offered a dangerous possibility for the corruption of the work of the Institute.[68] In 1937 Victor Kramer, son of a volunteer researcher at the Institute, published his Harvard A.B. thesis, *The National Institute of Health: A Study in Public Administration.* Dedicated to McCoy and acknowledged to be based on his interpretation, the thesis argued that if a director succeeded McCoy who desired rapid expansion and had "a flair for publicity," great harm "could be done to the Institute."[69] Scientists could be pressured, argued Kramer, to publish the results of their efforts prematurely, and fellowship donors might increasingly press for a greater determination of the type of research pursued. Referring to such a leader, Kramer said: "In this possibility together with the provisions . . . [of the Ransdell Act] there lies potential dynamite."[70]

Kramer published his study in 1937, just as Service leadership passed into hands that supported strongly the idea of expansion. Whether this was exploding dynamite or the irresistible wave of the future depended on the point of view of the observer. Surgeon General Cumming was replaced in 1936 by Thomas Parran. In 1937 the new Surgeon General reassigned McCoy to make a national survey of his special field of expertise, leprosy.[71] McCoy left the Service a year later to become director of the Department of Preventive Medicine and Public Health of the Louisiana State University Medical School in New Orleans. His position as director of the Institute had been merged in an internal reorganization with that of director of the Division of Scientific Research. The chief of that division, Assistant Surgeon General L. R. Thompson, became the new director of the Institute.

The shift to these new leaders was not as abrupt as it appeared on the surface. Both had been advocating a more active role for the Service for some time, and both were more congenial to the ideas of the New Deal than were their predecessors. Thomas Parran, "a fairly small man with a blonde face and red nose," had demonstrated imaginative leadership throughout his career in the Service.[72] A descendant of physicians from Calvert County, Maryland, Parran took his B.A. degree at St. Johns College in 1911 and had planned to attend the Johns Hopkins University Medical School.[73] Because of family financial constraints, however, the young man attended Georgetown University Medical School where he worked during the summers for Joseph J. Kinyoun, the founder of the Hygienic Laboratory who was then head of the District of Columbia Health Department Laboratory. Speaking of his relationship with Kinyoun, Parran later said, "I consider him to have been the first teacher I ever had and one who really determined my choice of public health as a career."[74] After receiving his M.D. *cum laude* from Georgetown in 1915, Parran completed an internship at Sibley Memorial Hospital in Washington, D.C., and accepted in 1916 a temporary appointment to do rural sanitation work for the Public Health Service. The following year he became a commissioned officer.

Parran took the Hygienic Laboratory course of instruction in laboratory methods in 1923. In 1926 he was appointed Assistant Surgeon General in charge of the Venereal Disease Division. In 1930 Franklin Roosevelt, then governor of New York, requested President Hoover to grant Parran a leave of absence to become state health officer for New York. In this capacity Parran developed a friendship with the governor and Mrs. Roosevelt that, after Roosevelt's election to the Presidency in 1932, gave Parran the "keys to the White House."[75]

According to Parran himself, he was asked to assume the office of

Surgeon General shortly after Roosevelt took the oath of office.[76] He declined the offer because of his friendship with Hugh Cumming. By the time the veteran Cumming's fourth term as Surgeon General ended in 1936, however, the pressure for change was such that Cumming stepped down, retiring with many honors.

One of Parran's major philosophical supporters within the Service was Assistant Surgeon General Lewis Ryers "Jimmie" Thompson, who had guided much of the discussion at the first meeting of the National Advisory Health Council in 1931.[77] Appointed director of the Division of Scientific Research in 1930, Thompson also saw the opportunity for expansion under the New Deal. He wrote to Parran in August 1933: "Personally I believe the time is ripe for us to produce a sound policy in public health for the future—it has been our one greatest trouble in the past and we are going to be left at the post if we can't meet changing conditions."[78]

Both Thompson and Parran were sympathetic to the goals of the national health movement. At a meeting with some of the movement's supporters in early 1933, Parran had remarked optimistically, "If the present upturn in business continues, with social planning an accepted part of the program, it should be appropriate within the next few months to present a real national health plan."[79] This broad plan included many items such as compulsory national health insurance that were ultimately defeated, but the longstanding proposal for consolidation of federal health agencies was finally achieved under Parran.

In January 1932 Parran had begun working on organizational charts of existing federal health activities and a proposal for consolidation at the request of then President-elect Roosevelt.[80] Parran included a chart of President Hoover's proposed reorganization, which placed agencies for health, education, and recreation under an assistant secretary for education, health, and recreation in the Interior Department. Parran's plan, however, made the Surgeon General of the Public Health Service effectively an assistant secretary in the Interior Department. All public health agencies were to be transferred into the Service, which would be reorganized into three categories: Health Protection, Medical Care, and the National Institute of Health. The Institute was to have jurisdiction over field research, a separate division to regulate biologic products, and its own in-house research.

The reorganization did not take place until 1939, but in that year the Service was transferred into the newly created Federal Security Agency. Other health bureaus transferred into this agency in 1939 or shortly thereafter included the Bureau of Vital Statistics, the Food and Drug Administration, and the Children's Bureau—all agencies proposed for consolidation into such a department by the national health movement. In 1953 these bureaus in the Federal Security Agency became the "Health" branch of the Department of Health, Education & Welfare, a department having a secretary in the president's cabinet.[81] Eighty years after the American Public Health Association had called for the creation of a cabinet-level national department of health, the United States finally adopted one formally.

Both Parran and Thompson had also envisioned a larger role for the National Institute of Health shortly after its creation than had Surgeon General Cumming and George McCoy. Cumming had appointed Parran and Thompson to a board in 1930 to consider the site of the new facilities authorized under the Ransdell Act.[82] Assistant Surgeon General John Kerr was also appointed, but McCoy was designated a "special consultant" to be called only if the board desired. At its first meeting this board displayed a marked shift in attitude about the potential for growth of the Institute. Writing to a friend about the board's recommendations, Cumming stated: "Much to my surprise and consternation, the members of the Board seemed to feel that unless we could get thirty acres [adjacent to the present site], we had better decide to move to a new location. To my mind, this amount of land is now and will be within the next fifteen or twenty years entirely unnecessary."[83]

Treasury Secretary Andrew Mellon agreed with Cumming, and the board revised its recommendation. Parran suggested, however, that a caveat be added so that the board could go on record concerning its analysis of the probable future needs of the Institute. He suggested a "safe-guarding" clause that stated: "It is difficult to dictate the full extent to which this Institute will develop, since this is dependent upon the amount of future activities and congressional appropriations, but it is likely that the 15 acre tract will need to be enlarged in the future to meet the probable growth of the Institute."[84]

Two new buildings, one for administration and one for laboratories, were constructed on the Twenty-fifth and E Streets, Northwest, campus.[85] They were not occupied until 1933, but in 1935 Thompson promoted a plan to rebuild the entire Institute on a forty-five acre tract of land in Bethesda, Maryland. Mr. and Mrs. Luke I. Wilson— he was associated with the Wilson Sporting Goods Company in Chicago and she was the daughter of one of the founders of the Woodward and Lothrop Department Store in Washington, D.C.—offered to donate their suburban estate to the government, "provided a use could be found for it which was of some general benefit to the people of the United States."[86] Thompson, who had been seeking land for the construction of an animal farm for the Institute, seized the opportunity to propose rebuilding of the entire facility. Cumming, who "considered other building programs of the Service of more importance," and McCoy, who reputedly also opposed the expansionist program, were at odds with the suggestion.[87] Cumming's retirement in 1936 cleared the way for the move, and Parran's friendship with the president and the secretary of the Treasury assisted the passage of the needed appropriation through Congress.[88] In 1937 Parran reorganized the research division of the Service, installing Thompson as director of the Institute and removing McCoy. An era of Public Health Service leadership had ended and a new one had begun.

It was not in buildings and acreage alone, however, that Parran and Thompson sought expansion. In 1934 Thompson arranged with Karl T. Compton, chairman of the newly created President's Science Advisory Board, for the board to study the state of medical research in the Public Health Service. Hoping for a recommendation that research should be expanded, Thompson also pushed to ensure that the subcommittee making the study would be staffed with friends of the Service. He achieved this goal: the members appointed were Surgeon General Parran, former director of the Hygienic Laboratory Milton Rosenau, and Rockefeller Institute director Simon Flexner. Not surprisingly, this subcommittee called for increased research in the chronic diseases and suggested that "funds for the scientific work of the Public Health Service . . . be increased by the sum of $2,500,000 over and above the allotment for 1934–35."[89] Furthermore, the dispersion of the funds was to be left to the discretion of the Surgeon General with the approval of the National Advisory Health Council.

This strong endorsement of research in the Public Health Service, coupled with a letter-writing campaign to win public and congressional support, bore fruit in 1935 with the passage of the Social Security Act. Under Title VI of that measure, the Service was authorized to spend $2 million annually on scientific research. And although Congress consistently refused to appropriate the maximum amount during the 1930s, the National Institute of Health did receive increased monies with which to expand research into chronic diseases. It was not until 1939, however, that expansion of the kind recommended in 1931 — the creation of new divisions at the Institute — was financially possible.

With this infusion of financial support, the Institute was able to expand a number of studies that had produced significant results, even under the economic constraints imposed by the Depression. Nutritional research, for instance, had revealed in 1931 that canned turnip greens were an excellent source of the then-still-unidentified vitamin that prevented pellagra.[90] Because of this finding, poor southern families — those in which the incidence of the disease was highest — were able to protect themselves with the inexpensive, readily available food.

Investigations into a variety of dental diseases were also conducted during the 1930s, most notably a long-term study on mottled tooth enamel initiated in 1931 by Institute researcher Trendley Dean.[91] This work eventually uncovered the beneficial effects of naturally occurring fluorides in preventing tooth decay.

Rickettsial disease research also expanded and produced significant results in the late 1930s. At the beginning of the decade, scientists in the Division of Pathology and Bacteriology confirmed that Rocky Mountain spotted fever, long thought confined to the Rocky Mountain region, existed in the eastern United States as well.[92] In 1931, moreover, they discovered that the vector of endemic typhus was the flea.[93] Intensive work on both of these diseases produced by 1937 a method for culturing rickettsiae in the yolk sacs of developing chick embryos, making possible the manufacture of an inexpensive vaccine.[94] Both the spotted fever and the typhus vaccines were widely used to protect United States troops during World War II.

In 1932 a section for the study of heart disease had been established at the Institute.[95] Under the direction of Assistant Surgeon General Arthur M. Stimson, this section worked on identifying the cause of rheumatic heart disease in its first five years. More extensive was the work of the cancer research program begun in 1922. Conducted cooperatively with the Department of Preventive Medicine and Hygiene at Harvard University, this program attacked cancer through fundamental studies along four major lines: research into the biological effects of radiation on malignant cells, studies of resistance and immunity to malignant growth, examinations of factors involved in the growth of normal and malignant cells, and research into the biochemistry of cancer cells.[96]

A flourishing program of cancer research was therefore in place when the National Cancer Institute was created in 1937. Further enhancing the commitment of the American people to medical research, the legislation that established the National Cancer Institute sped through Congress in record time and was sponsored by every senator.[97] This act included a provision for an extramural program— the awarding of grants to investigators at universities. The National Institute of Health had no such program, and, according to Donald C. Swain, Public Health Service officials were suspicious of such an undertaking.[98] The success of the Cancer Institute's extramural program and the experience of an even larger grants and contracts program during World War II, however, convinced Service leaders of the efficacy of both intramural and extramural research. The popularity of the categorical approach represented by the Cancer Institute, moreover, foreshadowed the creation of new categorical institutes after World War II.

By the mid-1940s, the position of the National Institute of Health within the federal government was secure and expanding. Under a sweeping reorganization act in 1944, a number of longstanding research goals were given the force of law.[99] Several provisions sought by Herty and Ransdell, which had been deleted from the National Institute of Health bill in order to accommodate political reality in the 1920s, were achieved without opposition in 1944. For example, the act authorized research fellowships with the specific goal of procuring "the most brilliant and promising research fellows from the United States and abroad." It also authorized fellowship recipients to be appointed "without regard for the civil-service laws" and compensated "without regard to the Classification Act of 1923." An extramural grants program was established for areas of medical research in addition to cancer. The mandate of the National Institute of Health, which was made a coequal branch of the Service with the Bureau of Medical Services and the Bureau of State Services, was worded in 1944 as an umbrella authorization that embraced both basic and applied investigations inside and outside the federal government. The act stated:

> The Surgeon General shall conduct in the Service, and encourage, cooperate with, and render assistance to other appropriate public authorities, scientific institutions, and scientists in the conduct of, and promote the coordination of, research, investigations, experiments, demonstrations, and studies relating to the causes, diagnosis, treatment, control, and prevention of physical and mental diseases and impairments of man, including water purification, sewage treatment, and pollution of lakes and streams.[100]

With the ascendancy of Thomas Parran and others who shared his views, the National Institute of Health had begun an expansion that saw the creation of eleven categorical institutes by the mid-1980s, an enormous extramural grants program, and the assumption of leadership in the world biomedical community. Although the size and scope of these developments were unprecedented, they were not created from whole cloth. The heritage of research tied to practical public health concerns has mingled with the emphasis on basic research that emerged after World War I to produce the unique configuration displayed by the National Institutes of Health in the last decades of the twentieth century.

Epilogue

A Century of Science for Health

The National Institutes of Health are a brilliant jewel
in the crown of HEW.
Wilbur J. Cohen, 1968

I n the half century that has elapsed since 1937, the National
Institutes of Health (NIH) have become the foremost biomedical
research facility not only in the United States but in the world.
The initiation and expansion of a program of grants have made
scientists in all states of the Union a part of the NIH community.
Furthermore, international grants, fellowships, exchanges, and col-
laborations have extended the NIH scientific web around the globe.
The story of this fifty years of mushrooming expansion is far too
complex to be written in one volume, let alone one chapter.[1] As the
NIH prepares to celebrate in 1987 the centennial of the Hygienic
Laboratory, however, it is instructive to consider the development of
the mature Institutes in light of their historical antecedents.

The National Institute of Health emerged from both the public health
and the scientific research communities. Until the end of World War
II, the Institute's public health roots clearly exerted the greatest impact on research priorities. Although a significant number of basic
studies were undertaken during this time, most of the Institute's
research was motivated either by requests from states for help in
public health emergencies or by problems relating to the Institute's
mandate to regulate biologicals. The list of such work is long; a few
examples suggest its nature: Joseph Kinyoun's study of contaminated
water wells in the District of Columbia; Milton J. Rosenau and John
Anderson's work on anaphylaxis; Joseph Goldberger's research on
pellagra in the southern United States; Trendly Dean's discovery of
the anticavity property of fluoride; and Roscoe R. Spencer and Ralph
R. Parker's development of a vaccine for Rocky Mountain spotted
fever. By the end of World War II, however, it had become clear that

chronic disease problems, especially cancer and heart disease, would not yield to short-term, on-site research. To combat these disorders, the basic science base on which applications could be built needed to be expanded, just as it had been in the century preceding the bacteriological "revolution" of the 1870s.

This conviction, put forth a generation earlier by scientists promoting cooperative research after World War I, became effectively translated into federal policy after World War II. In 1945 Vannevar Bush, director of the wartime Office of Scientific Research and Development, wrote a report requested by President Franklin Delano Roosevelt entitled *Science—The Endless Frontier.* It called for large-scale federal support for scientific research and embodied faith in the unlimited promise of science to improve the human condition.[2] Bush's report was followed by another, popularly known as the Steelman Report, which attempted to define the different types of research and appropriate federal involvement in each.[3] Within the Public Health Service, the National Institute of Health was assigned to work on basic problems, and the newly created Communicable Disease Center in Atlanta, Georgia, was given responsibility for applied work.[4] This decision altered the historic role of NIH researchers. The CDC took over their traditional responsibility for responding to epidemics and other health crises. No longer a secondary adjunct to applied public health measures, the NIH became an institution whose mission was entirely research—research through which, according to the convictions of Congress and the public, the medical "miracles" of the future would be uncovered. This differentiation of responsibilities within the Public Health Service was carried further in 1955, when the biologics control function of the NIH was placed in a separate division; in 1972, it became a bureau within the Food and Drug Administration.[5]

The shift in policy after World War II coincided with and, to some extent, was produced by efforts to create a national science policy, particularly a National Science Foundation. Not wishing to see biomedical research become one aspect of an umbrella science organization, NIH leaders moved aggressively to maintain the Institute's hegemony in medical research. Unfinished contracts for medical research let by the military services during the war were taken over by NIH, thus expanding its involvement with university researchers.[6] In addition, NIH leaders took advantage of public support for the creation of new institutes to study heart disease, mental health, and dental disease to expand the Institute's base. In 1948 Congress created the National Heart Institute and the National Institute of Dental Research and made the name of the National Institute of Health plural. The following year the National Institute of Mental Health also joined the NIH.[7] These new institutes had authority to make extramural grants, as did the existing National Cancer Institute, on whose successful program of awards the enabling legislation was modeled. Further expansion occurred during the directorships of Rolla Eugene Dyer and Henry Sebrell, when a clinical center was planned and constructed. In this new facility, NIH researchers could engage in clinical studies and enjoy onsite collaboration with their colleagues in basic science laboratories. Such an arrangement, envisioned in 1918 by chemist A. S. Loevenhart during the discussions about a proposed institute for chemo-medical research, became a reality in 1953.

This major transition, from a small intramural program to a large institution dealing with patients and forging a partnership with academia, revealed how significantly public attitudes had changed since the turn of the century. The arguments of Senator Joseph Ransdell, Charles Holmes Herty, and their supporters in the effort to enlarge basic biomedical research in the 1920s had contributed to the larger shift in public perception of the role of the federal government in such work. The 1920s were a "critical period," when attitudes changed slowly and new alliances were being formed. Events in the 1930s and 1940s accelerated this process and triggered the rapid expansion that occurred after World War II. During the Great Depression, the federal government took unprecedented actions to intervene in private affairs, providing economic, medical, educational, and other types of support under President Roosevelt's New Deal programs. The falling rates of return on investments, moreover, forced many philanthropic organizations into bankruptcy and severely curtailed the largesse of all. The ability of privately funded foundations to bear the cost of supporting biomedical research had been strained already in the 1920s; when the Depression further eroded their capacity to fund promising investigations, it became clear that private efforts would not be adequate to support science on a large scale.

The great achievements in science during World War II also enhanced public belief that scientific research offered an endless frontier on which a happier, healthier life could be built. The awesome achievements of the physicists in the Manhattan Project in creating an atomic bomb demonstrated what a concentrated effort on a broad basic science foundation could produce. Radar, developed for the war effort, provided the postwar world with an indispensable tool for effective civilian air traffic control. The introduction of penicillin, the first effective antibiotic, was followed by an organized and successful search for other antibiotics such as streptomycin.[8] Simultaneously with these achievements, military medical officers during the war delivered medical care of an unprecedented quality. Sulfonamides, penicillin, chloroquine to treat malaria, banks of whole blood and plasma, and, in trauma units, increased knowledge about shock—all of these were products of research since World War I that reduced casualties in World War II.[9] Having received excellent care during their tours of duty, soldiers returning to civilian life were not inclined to lower their expectations of quality.

In the postwar United States, chronic diseases, particularly cancer, supplanted epidemic maladies as the principal diseases feared by the public. With memories of wartime mobilization fresh in their minds, many people believed that chronic diseases could be brought under control if they were approached in the same manner as wartime emergencies. To this end, public advocates for medical research proposed a "fight on cancer," which received broad popular support. "To assemble the nation's scientific skill in a campaign against such an enemy," James Harvey Young has written, "came to seem a public policy with very high priority."[10]

Because the administrations of Harry Truman and Dwight D. Eisenhower focused on other national concerns, however, Congress seized the initiative in health research. Congressional advocates of health, among whom Congressman John Fogarty and Senator Lister Hill became chief spokesmen, were even more favorably inclined toward increasing health research expenditures, because other routes to improving the nation's health seemed blocked. From the end of the war until the mid-1960s, the American Medical Association strongly and consistently opposed health programs such as national health insurance schemes and federal aid to the elderly and indigent. Medical research, then, was the principal way by which congressmen could vote to improve their constituents' health.[11]

Private citizens supported congressional advocacy for health research; most notable was Mary Lasker, who had large financial resources, experience in public relations, and powerful connections. The efforts of these citizens to educate the public and dramatize health problems buttressed Congress's position. As Stephen Strickland has noted, this combination of lay and congressional forces joined with NIH and Public Health Service leaders to gain increased appropriations of up to 25 percent per year for the National Institutes of Health by the mid-1950s.[12]

Presiding over this expansion of basic biomedical research in the federal government was James A. Shannon, the NIH director appointed in 1955. A new breed of NIH director, Shannon had not come up through the Public Health Service ranks like his predecessors. Instead of quarantine assignments for the Service, Shannon had taught in the department of physiology at New York University College of

Medicine and directed research at the university's Goldwater Memorial Hospital. During World War II, he played a prominent role in malaria control research, receiving the Presidential Medal of Merit for his work. After the war he served as the director of the Squibb Institute for Medical research before coming to the NIH as associate director in charge of research for the newly created National Heart Institute. In 1952 he became associate director for the NIH and served in that capacity for three years before being named director.[13]

Under Shannon, the NIH enjoyed what are fondly remembered as its Golden Years. The total NIH budget, $29 million in 1948 and $98 million when Shannon took office, rose to $1.4 billion by 1967. During this same period, 1948 to 1967, the proportion of the budget expended in research, training, and construction grants rose from 54 percent to 75 percent.[14] Foreign research grants increased from 5 awards worth $130,000 in 1947 to 981 worth $14,956,000 in 1963, the peak year for these awards.[15] Such expenditures produced results: by 1983 over eighty Nobel laureates in "Chemistry" or in "Physiology or Medicine" had conducted at least a part of their research with NIH support. Four of these scientists did their prizewinning research on the NIH campus in Bethesda. These intramural NIH laureates enlarged our knowledge of the genetic code that governs life processes, helped to elucidate the metabolic processes within the body, examined the chemistry of nerve transmission, and investigated so-called slow virus diseases.[16] Inspired by the outstanding records of NIH scientists, Wilbur J. Cohen, then secretary of the Department of Health, Education & Welfare (HEW), declared in 1968: "The National Institutes of Health are a brilliant jewel in the crown of HEW."[17]

In addition to basic research advances, many diagnostic techniques, innovative therapies, and preventive measures were developed by NIH researchers and grantees throughout the 1950s and 1960s. The National Cancer Institute, for example, tested some eighty-five thousand women in a clinical trial of the diagnostic procedure developed by George N. Papanicolaou—popularly known as the "Pap test"—which provided quick, painless, and inexpensive diagnosis of cervical cancer at an early, treatable stage.[18] Scientists associated with the National Institute of Arthritis and Metabolic Diseases conducted research and testing that led to oral substitutes for insulin in the treatment of diabetes.[19] Grantees of the National Heart Institute pioneered in the 1950s new methods in open heart surgery now widely used to save lives, such as hypothermia techniques, the heart-lung machine, and blood vessel grafting.[20] Research leading to a vaccine against one of the most widespread childhood diseases, measles, was supported by the National Institute of Allergy and Infectious Diseases.[21]

These few examples illustrate the practical results derived from dollars invested in health research. Unfortunately for the NIH, however, most medical breakthroughs were identified with a particular investigator and his or her home institution rather than with the federal agency that provided funding for the research. None of these advances in basic or applied science, moreover, entirely eliminated cancer, which was the foremost dread disease, or heart disease, or a host of other ills that flesh is heir to. Further, basic science had become so complex that much of this research was difficult for any nonscientist to comprehend. To many people, it seemed that the public was being asked to support the scientific enterprise largely on faith. During the Golden Years, public confidence in science remained strong. This salubrious situation changed in the late 1960s for a variety of reasons.

Paul Starr, in *The Social Transformation of American Medicine*, identified three phases in postwar medical policy in the United States. The first, which coincided with the Golden Years, favored the growth of medical research and hospital construction without disturbing the fee-for-service organization of private medical practitioners. The second, beginning during the liberal years of the mid-sixties, focused on the extension of primary medical care to the disadvantaged. Bills establishing Medicare and Medicaid were enacted. By the early 1970s, however, inflation began to affect the United States economy seriously, in part because of the "guns and butter" policies of the Johnson administration during the Vietnam war. Medical costs, in particular, seemed to be rising uncontrollably. Public demand that the costs of federal programs be controlled soon outweighed all earlier concerns.[22] The NIH did not escape the impact of this larger trend.

In the 1960s the Lasker forces and other citizens' lobbies began to insist that the NIH produce therapeutic results after twenty years of investment in basic science. The disaffection of such groups marked the beginning of a breakdown in the powerful postwar coalition of Congress, lay advocates, and NIH leadership that had achieved such rapid growth in health research. Further eroding the once powerful "health syndicate" was the retirement of Lister Hill from the Senate and Congressman John Fogarty's death. Demands that NIH become more relevant to questions of health care delivery also increased throughout the second half of the 1960s. As Shannon prepared to retire as NIH director in 1968, one writer noted:

Stated oversimply, in the debate over the government's health activities there are, at one extreme, those who contend that NIH, under Shannon, has evolved into an organization that is concerned with science rather than with sick people and, at the other pole, those who contend that the first view is preposterous—that basic science, as supported and conducted by NIH, is the *sine qua non* of the therapies that are impatiently called for by the advocates of improved medical service.[23]

In response to such criticism, Congress directed NIH to establish Regional Medical Programs whose purpose was to make research findings available to the practicing physician as soon as possible. Other initiatives, such as the high blood pressure education program begun in 1971, encouraged not only physicians but also the public to act on knowledge gained in the laboratory.[24] In addition, the National Library of Medicine became a component part of the NIH. This expanded library, which had begun as the library of the Surgeon General of the Army under John Shaw Billings, developed into the foremost biomedical communications center in the world. Its on-line data bases, accessible to scientists across the United States and in many foreign countries, make the contents of *Index Medicus* and a number of other scientific bibliographies instantly available from computer terminals.[25]

Another criticism of the Institutes that originated in the liberal period of the 1960s focused on the management of the extramural grants program. Grant awards were made by a two-tiered review system. The first level of review was vested in "study sections," groups of nongovernmental scientists convened to evaluate the scientific merits of proposals and to recommend the best for funding. Institute Advisory Councils, composed of physicians, scientists, and informed laypersons, constituted the second level of review. In the early sixties, it was noted that grant awards were concentrated primarily in a few institutions.[26] This situation produced charges of possible conflicts of interest, cronyism, and elitism—serious allegations in a democratic society traditionally suspicious of special interest groups. In response to this and to later attacks on the peer review system, the NIH instituted some changes, but it resisted any pressures to award grants on a balanced geographic basis instead of on scientific merit. In 1974 Robert S. Stone, then NIH director, tersely stated the philosophy of the Institutes: "Science is intrinsically elitist in that it must strive for excellence in the employment of human talent. . . . In the case of government supported science, the presumption is that the taxpayer does not want to pay for mediocrity."[27]

With the advent of the Nixon administration, both the expansion of the Golden Years and the emphasis of the 1960s on equality and democratization within government gave way to increasing concern over economic problems in American society. As inflation seemed to spiral endlessly upward, Congress was pressed to control costs in government. The Nixon administration moved aggressively to curtail some programs, even impounding funds appropriated by Congress. The number of research grants awarded by the NIH was reduced; training grants for young researchers were virtually eliminated; and the number of intramural NIH positions restricted.[28] Presidential and congressional desire to receive tangible results for tax revenues expended also helped to promote "targeted" research projects at the expense of open-ended basic research. A "War on Cancer," declared in 1971, greatly expanded all aspects of research in the National Cancer Institute, especially efforts to find specific chemotherapies.[29] The status of the Cancer Institute within the NIH also changed; its director became a presidential appointee, and its budget had to be transmitted to the President's Office of Management and Budget without change by NIH or HEW.

The scientific community reacted strongly to these developments, believing Congress to be encroaching on the decisions best made by scientists. "Acceptance of whatever the legislative juggernaut demands seems inevitable," wrote one critic. "Much of the freedom of science is now being legislated away and we are approaching the Russian system of directed research."[30] Other scientists predicted accurately that the public would become disillusioned with science if targeted research programs did not provide a quick victory over cancer.[31] The longstanding fear of the scientific community, so much in evidence in the early twentieth century, that government patronage of science would perforce lead to government control, seemed menacingly evident in 1972.

Another indication of the increasing politicization of biomedical science during the Nixon era was a rapid turnover in NIH directors. Previously an internal Public Health Service position, the NIH directorship became a presidential appointment in 1971 under the Cancer Act. Robert Q. Marston, who succeeded James A. Shannon as director in 1968, served only through President Richard M. Nixon's first term; he was replaced by Robert S. Stone in 1973.[32] Stone, who reportedly was chosen because his loyalty to the philosophy of the Nixon administration exceeded that to NIH, was dismissed after serving little more than a year, presumably because he changed his mind.[33] He was succeeded in 1975 by Donald S. Fredrickson, a longtime member of the NIH community. Fredrickson's six-year tenure until he retired in 1981 seemed to return a sense of stability to the head office.

The Advisory Councils of the Institutes were also touched by this trend. Pressures to appoint members whose politics agreed with those of the incumbent administration threatened to trivialize the stature of these councils. People feared that Advisory Councils would become mere rubber stamps for presidential directives, a sorry state for these bodies, whose distinguished earlier members included such notables in early scientific medicine as William H. Welch.[34]

One other target of those promoting tight management policies was the heart of the extramural program—the system of grants-in-aid. Unlike the 1960s, when the allocation of grants was questioned, budget-conscious planners in the 1970s looked searchingly at the concept of grants as an instrument to foster research. Proponents of applied research argued that much biomedical research could be done under contracts such as those used by the military and space agencies.[35] David Schwartzman, an economics professor in the New School for Social Research, argued similarly that the empirical methods of industry—the type of research generally supported by contracts rather than grants—had "proved to be a much better source of useful drugs than had basic research in the pure sciences. In fact," he went on, "spinoffs from industry's empirical approach had profited basic science theory more than had that theory contributed to practical drug discovery."[36]

With its quid pro quo nature, the contract provided strict accountability for the expenditure of public revenues. Researchers in basic science, however, cannot describe at the outset what conclusions will be reached during a given period of time. Because of this, the more flexible instrument of the grant-in-aid is preferred by scientists. Debates over these two types of funding for biomedical research highlighted traditional tensions between Congress, with its oversight responsibilities for all federal programs, however complex, and the biomedical research community, which requires great freedom to pursue scientific leads as they occur.

The basic science community, which had enjoyed public faith for so long, was unprepared to do major battle over these issues in the political arena. Medical schools came to the defense of the NIH only after the Nixon administration sharply curtailed training grants for medical students and impounded funds for research grants.[37] The initial public response of the NIH community to the political and economic changes, moreover, appeared to be self-serving in its arguments. Insistence on the independence of NIH from congressional and presidential intervention—often couched in terms such as the requirement of scientists for "tranquility in research"—was seen as "evidence of the arrogance of scientists who want public money without public accountability."[38]

Since the end of World War II, furthermore, the basic science community had rarely attempted to educate the public through books and articles on the relationship between basic research and long-term medical advances. As early as 1966 a deputy director of the President's

Office of Science and Technology warned: "We must cease to give the impression that we don't have time to talk to the public—and even worse that if we did talk to them, they couldn't grasp our meaning anyway."[39] When reductions in the budget became a reality several years later, a few studies of this nature were produced, most notably J. H. Comroe and R. D. Dripps's 1974 article, "Ben Franklin and Open-Heart Surgery."[40] Clearly, if NIH hoped to recover the broad support it had enjoyed in the Golden Years, its leaders would have to give increasing attention to communication with its constituents.

With the changes introduced in the 1970s and brought about by many factors in the larger society, the eleven Institutes that today compose the NIH find themselves competing for limited federal resources with sister agencies. NIH director James B. Wyngaarden observed in 1983 that in the context of the present economy, the NIH "has been well treated by the Administration and the Congress, but it cannot anticipate extraordinary growth in the foreseeable future. In my view," he said, "we are facing more than a temporary funding constraint in biomedical science; rather, we have entered a new steady state that all of us, NIH and universities alike, would do well to view as the future norm."[41] In order to maintain its position in the allocation of federal resources, according to one recommendation made in a study of the Institutes in 1984, the NIH needed to strengthen its public information program because there was little evidence that the public was aware of its work.[42] The need for public support in order to succeed in the bureaucratic competition for scarce funds was a reality that the Public Health Service knew well early in its history.

The tight budget situation in the 1980s is little different from that experienced by the Hygienic Laboratory in the early twentieth century. A more significant question for the future of the NIH is the extent to which Congress, in response to pressure from a variety of groups, will attempt to direct the course of research in the Institutes. Mandates to spend money on particular diseases at the expense of basic studies relevant to all disease problems are always a difficult problem for the NIH. In response to public fear about Acquired Immune Deficiency Syndrome, for example, NIH researchers and their counterparts in France began an intensive study of the disease and identified a virus suspected to be the causative agent. NIH researchers, moreover, developed a screening test for blood donors to protect the nation's blood supply from contamination with the AIDS virus. AIDS was perceived to be a major threat to public health, and because of previous basic research in virology and immunology, the Institutes were able to make rapid progress in understanding this disease.[43]

In contrast, pressures from many public groups to study particular diseases or to establish new institutes have been viewed as unproductive for the long range. According to Wyngaarden, such directed research has "adverse effects on administrative costs and flexibility" and establishes compartmentalization "that is counter to the direction in which science is moving."[44] Within the Institutes, some study has been done in examining the balance between basic and applied research. One of these studies concluded that "scientific knowledge and discoveries come from many sources, by often unforeseen routes, and that we still know far too little about the course and determinants of those research processes that may variously result in therapeutic innovation or in fundamental knowledge."[45]

One thing that has been discerned is that biomedical science of both types is being done increasingly by Ph.D. specialists and less by researchers with M.D. degrees. There are a number of reasons for this shift. The professionalization of research and the need for highly specialized skills has militated against the clinically trained physician. The severe curtailment of training grants also has had an impact on medical students contemplating research careers. Without assistance, few of them are willing to assume the burden of repaying large medical school debts from a researcher's salary instead of from the more comfortable position of a private practitioner. And yet, as Wyngaarden has noted, in biomedical research the "trained clinical investigator is the critical link between the laboratory and the health care provider."[46]

Throughout these public debates on budgets and policy, the NIH has maintained its emphasis on scientific excellence, a priority that has been its hallmark since 1902 when the Hygienic Laboratory expanded beyond a single permanent staff member.[47] In addition to continued support of basic biomedical research, however, the Institutes have expanded their scope to include more public involvement. In 1975, for instance, the *Journal of the American Medical Association* began publishing a column, "Notes from the NIH," which reported research results applicable to clinical practice. A series of lectures, Medicine for the Layman, was also inaugurated to interpret research findings for nonscientist citizens. An enlarged public education program has produced a wealth of pamphlets available to the public on topics from child development to the medical problems of the elderly. Consensus Development Conferences, which are meetings of specialists in particular disease problems, regularly produce statements that interpret the findings of clinical trials and evaluate treatment methods.[48] An Ambulatory Care Research Facility has been added to the Clinical Center on the Bethesda campus in order to expand the Institutes's capacity for clinical research. It will likely also serve as a model for delivering excellent medical care on an outpatient basis, a change in

American health care patterns that, it is hoped, will hold down the cost of being sick.

Some of these changes, all of which have reemphasized the public health roots of the NIH, have brought the Institutes into contact with the larger questions of medical economics and biomedical ethics. In relation to the latter, public concern in the last two decades about the use of humans in testing new drugs, especially in cancer chemotherapy, produced guidelines for the use of human subjects in all research projects. Similar questions about potential dangers in research on recombinant DNA—popularly known as genetic engineering—led the scientific community to request that NIH also formulate general guidelines for work in this area.[49]

Such difficult issues point up both the problems and the vastly expanded potential for further achievements in medical diagnosis and therapy by scientists using increasingly sophisticated technology and methods. Researchers in the National Institute of Dental Research and the National Institute of Allergy and Infectious Diseases, for example, have applied recombinant DNA techniques to produce a vaccine that protects mice from the herpes virus that plagues humans most commonly as cold sores, or "fever blisters," on the lips.[50] In addition, a promising type of membrane oxygenator being developed in the National Heart, Lung, and Blood Institute may enable physicians to provide respiratory assistance to patients for a week or more without damaging the lungs, which conventional respirators do over such long time periods.[51] Already, physicians employ CAT scanners and PET scanners to probe the mysteries of the soft tissues of the body. A new device, the nuclear magnetic resonance, or NMR, scanner, developed with NIH support, promises to yield even better information with no danger of radiation to the patient. Many scientists, in fact, believe that recent discoveries in basic science have ushered in a new Golden Age that may produce, among many other things, vaccines to prevent the worldwide scourge of malaria and effective medications for biochemically caused mental disorders.

The Bethesda campus of the Institutes is characterized by an informality and scientific camaraderie usually found on university campuses. Young researchers can approach Nobel laureates and receive immediate criticism and counsel on research problems. The cafeteria in the Clinical Center is populated with the white laboratory coats of clinicians and with people poring over computer printouts of data from experiments. The Journal Club, established by Milton Rosenau in 1902, has expanded into many journal clubs, which meet in each laboratory and have been exported to other laboratories throughout the world.[52]

In celebrating the centennial of Joseph Kinyoun's Hygienic Laboratory, the NIH selected "A Century of Science for Health" as the theme for the observance. Kinyoun would doubtless be astounded at the size and scope of NIH research today. Yet he, as well as those who argued in the early decades of the twentieth century for expansion in federal biomedical science, would likely be gratified by the contributions to human health fostered by this institution during its first century. As Kinyoun could not have predicted how his laboratory of hygiene would evolve, neither can we foresee the future of federal medical research. Richard Shryock, writing in 1947, noted that it would be a "bold prophet who would set limits to the future advance of medical science, provided society continues to support research."[53] That same observation holds true today: if the American people continue to make medical research a public priority and to place their faith in the National Institutes of Health as the principal federal agency to nurture promising investigations, it would be a bold prophet, indeed, who could forecast the bounds of discovery in federal biomedical research during the century ahead.

Notable Contributions of Public Health Service Scientists to 1940

This table is adapted from Jeanette Barry, comp., *Notable Contributions to Medical Research by Public Health Service Scientists: A Bibliography to 1940* (Washington, D.C.: Government Printing Office, 1960), pp. xi–xiv.

An asterisk (*) indicates that the person was starred in *American Men of Science*; an "S" indicates that the person was the recipient of the Sedgwick Memorial Medal of the American Public Health Association. The table is arranged chronologically by years of service in the Public Health Service (PHS).

Service in PHS	Name	Areas of Contribution
1890–1909 * S	Rosenau, Milton J. (1869–1946) Epidemiologist	Anaphylaxis; typhoid studies; standardization of biological products; text: *Preventive Medicine and Hygiene*
1898–1915	Anderson, John F. (1871–1958) Bacteriologist	*Dermacentor andersoni* (Stiles); measles transmitted to monkeys; test for typhus; anaphylaxis and allergy; first use of word *allergin*
1899–1929 *	Goldberger, Joseph (1874–1929) Bacteriologist and epidemiologist	"Straw itch" (Dermatitis schambergi); transmission of typhus by lice; experimental production of pellagra and prevention by proper diet

Service in PHS	Name	Areas of Contribution
1900–1938 *	Francis, Edward (1872–1957) Bacteriologist	"Tularemia Francis" (Deer-fly fever); operative procedure in embalming; agar as culture medium
1900–1938	McCoy, George W. (1876–1952) Bacteriologist, immunologist, and epidemiologist	Isolation of *Bacterium tularense*; plague in California ground squirrels; leprosy—epidemiology and public health management
1902–31	Stiles, C. W. (1876–1941) Zoologist	Hookworm identification and control in North America; *Index-Catalog of Medical and Veterinary Zoology*
1902–41	Stimson, A. M. (1876–1953) Bacteriologist and epidemiologist	*Leptospira icterohaemorrhagiae*; modification of Pasteur rabies treatment and method for vaccine preparation; identification of rabies vaccine reactions
1903–29 * S	Frost, Wade Hampton (1880–1938) Epidemiologist	Epidemiological method; stream pollution studies
1904–13 *	Hunt, Reid (1870–1948) Pharmacologist	Discovery of thyroid hormone in blood; Hunt's reaction: acetonitrile test for thyroid; toxicity of alcohol; hypotensive effect of acetylcholine
1905–9 *	Kastle, Joseph H. (1864–1916) Chemist	Chemical tests for blood; Kastle's reagent; oxygen catalysts
1906–47	Schwartz, Louis (1883–1963) Dermatologist	Dermatitis and melanosis due to photosensitization
1907–39 *	Seidell, Atherton (1878–1961) Chemist	Chemistry of vitamins; concentration of antineuritic substances; solubility of organic and inorganic compounds; chemistry of thyroid, with Reid Hunt

Service in PHS	Name	Areas of Contribution
1908–9, 1917	Wherry, William B. (1874–1936) Bacteriologist	Discovery of sylvatic plague in California ground squirrels; tularemia in humans first identified
1909–45	Leake, James P. (1881–1973) Immunologist	Multiple pressure method of vaccination; poliomyelitis epidemiology
1913–43 *	Voegtlin, Carl (1879–1960) Chemist	Action of arsenicals
1914–47	Spencer, R. R. (1888–1982) Bacteriologist and immunologist	Development of Rocky Mountain spotted fever vaccine, with R. R. Parker
1916–46	Bengtson, Ida A. (1881–1952) Bacteriologist	New variety of *Clostridium botulinum* ("C"); standardization of gas gangrene antitoxins
1916–50 * S	Armstrong, Charles (1886–1967) Bacteriologist and pathologist	"Armstrong's disease" (Lymphocytic choriomeningitis); post-vaccinal tetanus; experimental transmission of poliomyelitis to animals; psittacosis
1916–50 * S	Dyer, Rollo E. (1886–1971) Pathologist and epidemiologist	"Murine typhus" (Endemic typhus)—transmission and vaccine; scarlet fever antitoxin
1918–45	Evans, Alice C. (1881–1975) Bacteriologist	Brucellosis; Evans salt solution; etiology of epidemic encephalitis; Evans modification
1920–27 *	Clark, William M. (1884–1964) Chemist	Acid-base equilibria; oxidation-reduction equilibria; hydrogen ion determination
1920–51	Smith, Maurice I. (1887–1951) Pharmacologist	Smith method of assaying ergonovine; Jamaica-ginger paralysis

Service in PHS	Name	Areas of Contribution
1921–29 S	Maxcy, Kenneth (1889–1966) Epidemiologist	"Maxcy's disease" (Endemic typhus)
1921–49	Parker, R. R. (1888–1949) Entomologist	Tularemia infection in ticks; development of Rocky Mountain spotted fever vaccine, with R. R. Spencer
1929–51 *	Hudson, Claude (1881–1952) Chemist	Structure of carbohydrates; anomerism; Hudson's lactone rule

Texts of the Ransdell and Parker Acts

Ransdell Act

An Act to establish and operate a National Institute of Health, to create a system of fellowships in said institute, and to authorize the Government to accept donations for use in ascertaining the cause, prevention, and cure of disease affecting human beings, and for other purposes. Public Law No. 251, 71st Congress, 2nd session, May 26, 1930.

Be it enacted by the Senate and House of Representatives of the United States of America in Congress assembled, That the Hygienic Laboratory of the Public Health Service shall hereafter be known as the National Institute of Health, and all laws, authorizations, and appropriations pertaining to the Hygienic Laboratory shall hereafter be applicable for the operation and maintenance of the National Institute of Health. The Secretary of the Treasury is authorized to utilize the site now occupied by the Hygienic Laboratory and the land adjacent thereto owned by the Government and available for this purpose, or when funds are available therefor, to acquire sites by purchase, condemnation, or otherwise, in or near the District of Columbia, and to erect thereon and to furnish and equip suitable and adequate buildings for the use of such institute. In the administration and operation of this institute the Surgeon General shall select persons who show unusual aptitude in science. There is hereby authorized to be appropriated, out of any money in the Treasury not otherwise appropriated, the sum of $750,000, or so much thereof as may be necessary for construction and equipment of additional buildings at the present Hygienic Laboratory of the Public Health Service, Washington, District of Columbia.

Sec. 2. The Secretary of the Treasury is authorized to accept on behalf of the United States gifts made unconditionally by will or otherwise for study, investigation, and research in the fundamental problems of the diseases of man and matters pertaining thereto, and for the acquisition of grounds or for the erection, equipment, and maintenance of buildings and premises: *Provided,*

That conditional gifts may be accepted if recommended by the Surgeon General and the National Advisory Health Council. Any such gifts shall be held in trusts and shall be invested by the Secretary of the Treasury in securities of the United States, and the principal or income thereof shall be expended by the Surgeon General, with the approval of the Secretary of the Treasury, for the purposes indicated in this act, subject to the same examination and audit as provided for appropriations made for the Public Health Service by Congress. Donations of $500,000 or over in aid of research will be acknowledged permanently by the establishment within the institute of suitable memorials to the donors. The Surgeon General, with the approval of the Secretary of the Treasury, is authorized to establish and maintain fellowships in the National Institute of Health, from funds donated for that purpose.

Sec. 3. Individual scientists, other than commissioned officers of the Public Health Service, designated by the Surgeon General to receive fellowships may be appointed for duty in the National Institute of Health established by this act. During the period of such fellowship these appointees shall hold appointments under regulations promulgated by the Secretary of the Treasury and shall be subject to administrative regulations for the conduct of the Public Health Service. Scientists so selected may likewise be designated for the prosecution of investigations in other localities and institutions in this and other countries during the term of their fellowships.

Sec. 4. The Secretary of the Treasury, upon the recommendation of the Surgeon General, is authorized (1) to designate the titles and fix the compensation of the necessary scientific personnel under regulations approved by the President; (2) in accordance with the civil service laws to appoint, and in accordance with the classification act of 1923, and amendments thereto, fix compensation of such clerical and other assistants; and (3) to make such expenditures (including expenditures for personal services and rent at the seat of government, for books of reference, periodicals, and exhibits, and for printing and binding) as he deems necessary for the proper administration of such institution.

Sec. 5. The facilities of the institute shall from time to time be made available to bona fide health authorities of States, counties, or municipalities for purposes of instruction and investigation.

Sec. 6. That hereafter the Director of the National Institute of Health while so serving shall have the rank and shall receive the pay and allowances of a medical director of the Public Health Service.

Parker Act

An Act to provide for the coordination of the pubic health activities of the Government, and for other purposes. Public Law No. 106, 71st Congress, 2nd session, April 9, 1930.

Be it enacted by the Senate and House of Representatives of the United States of America in Congress assembled, That upon the request of the head of an executive department or an independent establishment which is carrying on a public health activity the Secretary of the Treasury is authorized to detail officers or employees of the Public Health Service to such department or independent establishment in order to cooperate in such work. When officers or employees are so detailed their salaries and allowances shall be paid by the Public Health Service from applicable appropriations.

Sec. 2. (a) The Surgeon General of the Public Health Service is authorized to detail personnel of the Public Health Service to educational and research institutions for special studies of scientific problems relating to public health and for the dissemination of information relating to public health, and to extend the facilities of the Public Health Service to health officials and scientists engaged in special study.

(b) The Secretary of the Treasury is authorized to establish such additional divisions in the Hygienic Laboratory in the District of Columbia as he deems necessary to provide agencies for the solution of public health problems, and facilities therein for the coordination of research by public health officials and other scientists and for demonstrations of sanitary methods and appliances.

Sec. 3. The administrative office and bureau divisions of the Public Health Service in the District of Columbia shall be administered as a part of the departmental organization, and the scientific offices and research laboratories of the Public Health Service (whether or not in the District of Columbia) shall be administered as a part of the field service.

Sec. 4. Hereafter, under such regulations as the President may prescribe, medical, dental, sanitary engineer, and pharmacist officers selected for general service in the regular corps of the Public Health Service and subject to change of station shall be appointed by the President, by and with the advice and consent of the Senate; original appointments shall be made only in the grade corresponding to that of assistant surgeon or passed assistant surgeon, except as provided under sections 5 and 6 of this act.

Sec. 5. The President is authorized to appoint, by and with the advice and consent of the Senate, to grades in the regular corps not above that of medical director, under such regulations as he may prescribe, not to exceed a total of fifty-five medical, dental, sanitary engineer, and pharmacist officers in the Public Health Service upon the date of passage of this act (except commissioned officers of the regular corps). Not more than four such appointments shall be in a grade above that of surgeon. In making such appointments due regard shall be had the salary received by such officer at the time of such appointment. For purposes of pay and pay period, said officers shall be credited only with active service in the Public Health Service and active commissioned service in the Army and the Navy.

Sec. 6. The Secretary of the Treasury is authorized to order officers in the reserve of the Public Health Service to active duty for the purpose of training and of determining their fitness for appointment in the regular corps, and such active duty shall be credited for purposes of future promotion in the regular corps.

Sec. 7. Whenever commissioned officers of the Public Health Service are not available for the performance of permanent duties requiring highly specialized training and experience in scientific research, the Secretary of the Treasury shall report that fact to the President with his recommendations, and the President, under the provision of this section, is authorized to appoint, by and with the advice and consent of the Senate, not to exceed three persons in any one fiscal year to grades in the regular corps of the Public Health Service above that of assistant surgeon, but not to a grade above that of medical director; and for purposes of pay and pay period any person appointed under the provisions of this section shall be considered as having had on the date of appointment service equal to that of the junior officer of the grade to which appointed.

Sec. 8. Any person commissioned in the regular corps of the Public Health Service under the provisions of this act of an age greater than forty-five years, if placed on waiting orders for disability incurred in line of duty, shall receive pay at the rate of 4 per centum of active pay for each complete year of service in the Army, Navy, or Public Health Service, the total to be not more than 75 per centum.

Sec. 9. Hereafter commissioned officers of the regular corps of the Public Health Service, after examination under regulations approved by the President, shall be promoted according to the same length of service and shall receive the same pay and allowances as are now or may hereafter be authorized for officers of corresponding grades of the Medical Corps of the Army, except that—

(a) For purposes of future promotion an officer whose original appointment to the regular corps under the provisions of this act is in a grade above that of assistant surgeon shall be considered as having had on the date of appointment service equal to that of the junior officer of the grade to which appointed; if the actual service of such officer in the Public Health Service exceeds that of the junior officer of the grade, such actual service not exceeding ten years for a passed assistant surgeon, and fourteen years for a surgeon shall be credited for purposes of future promotion;

(b) Pharmacists shall not be promoted to the grade of passed assistant surgeon until after five years of service in the grade of assistant surgeon and shall not be promoted above the grade of passed assistant surgeon.

(c) When an officer, after examination under regulations approved by the President, is found not qualified for promotion for reasons other than physical disability incurred in line of duty—

(1) If in the grade of assistant surgeon, he shall be separated from the service and paid six months' pay and allowances;

(2) If in the grade of passed assistant surgeon, he shall be separated from the service and paid one year's pay and allowances; and

(3) If in the grade of surgeon or of senior surgeon, he shall be reported as not in line of promotion, or placed on waiting orders and paid at the rate of 2½ per centum for each complete year of active commissioned service in the Public Health Service, but in no case to exceed 60 per centum of his active pay at the time he is placed on waiting orders.

Sec. 10. (a) The President is authorized to prescribe appropriate titles for commissioned officers of the Public Health Service other than medical officers, corresponding to the grades of medical officers. Hereafter officers of the Public Health Service in the grade of Assistant Surgeon General (except those in charge of bureau divisions) shall be known and designated as medical directors. The limitation now imposed by law upon the number of senior surgeons and Assistant Surgeons General at large of the Public Health Service on active duty is hereby repealed.

(b) Hereafter the Surgeon General of the Public Health Service shall be entitled to the same pay and allowances as the Surgeon General of the Army; and a regular commissioned officer of the Public Health Service who serves as Surgeon General shall, upon the expiration of his commission, if not reappointed as Surgeon General, revert to the grade and number in the regular corps that he would have occupied had he not served as Surgeon General.

(c) The officer detailed as chief of the narcotics division of the Public Health Service shall, while thus serving, be an Assistant Surgeon General, subject to the provisions of law applicable to Assistant Surgeons General in charge of other administrative divisions of the Public Health Service.

Sec. 11. Hereafter the Secretary of the Treasury shall appoint, in accordance with the civil service laws, all officers and employees, other than commissioned officers, of the Public Health Service, and may make any such appointment effective as of the date on which the officer or employee enters upon duty: *Provided*, That any regulations which may be prescribed as to the qualifications as to the appointment of medical officers or employees shall give no preference to any school of medicine.

Sec. 12. Hereafter officers of the Public Health Service when disabled on account of sickness or injury incurred in line of duty shall be entitled to medical, surgical, and hospital services and supplies under such regulations as the Secretary of the Treasury may prescribe.

Sec. 13. Hereafter the advisory board for the Hygienic Laboratory shall be known as the National Advisory Health Council, and the Surgeon General of the Public Health Service, with the approval of the Secretary of the Treasury, is authorized to appoint, from representatives of the public health profession, five additional members of such council. The terms of service, compensation, and allowances of such additional members shall be the same as the other members of such council not in the regular employment of the Government, except that the terms of service of the members first appointed shall be so arranged that the terms of not more than two members shall expire each year. Such council, in addition to its other function, shall advise the Surgeon General of the Public Health Service in respect to public health activities.

Note on Sources

The establishment of the National Institute of Health (NIH) in 1930 was one instance of the increasing federalization of science in the early twentieth century. Studying the many factors involved in the creation of such an institution leads one to a wide variety of primary and secondary sources that shed light on how federal policy is made. Policy is ultimately developed by the decisions of individuals, of course, and a number of private collections of papers were rich sources for analyzing the actions and beliefs of people who played a major role in the shaping of research policy in these years of change. Two collections in particular were exceptionally valuable. The Charles Holmes Herty Papers at Emory University provided almost day-by-day documentation of efforts by Herty and Senator Joseph E. Ransdell to enlarge federal support for biomedical research. Dr. Herty was a prolific correspondent with many people who played key roles in this area in the 1920s. Archivist Monica J. Blanchard provided convenient access to the 153 manuscript boxes with her excellent descriptive inventory, *Guide to the Charles Holmes Herty Papers* (Atlanta: Special Collections Department, Robert W. Woodruff Library for Advanced Studies, Emory University, 1981). Before the inventory was published, moreover, she served as a walking index for locating particular letters.

The Hugh Smith Cumming Papers in the Manuscripts Department, Alderman Library, the University of Virginia, were also a rich source of information about the Surgeon General himself, internal affairs of the Public Health Service, and major figures in the medical community. I am indebted to Dr. Cumming's son, Ambassador Hugh S. Cumming, Jr., who allowed me access to the restricted portions of his father's papers.

The Joseph Eugene Ransdell Papers at the Louisiana State University Library Archives in Baton Rouge contained a few interesting documents relating to the Conference Board of the National Institute of Health and the National Health Council. Overall, the collection is small and unrewarding. Two volumes of memoirs prepared by Assistant Surgeon General John W. Kerr provided insight into the work of the Service and the development of scientific research during his tenure as director of the Division of Scientific Research. Dr. Kerr's daughter, Helen Pratt Kerr Grismer, kindly allowed me to inspect these manuscripts, which are held by her family.

The Thomas Parran Papers, which were in the process of being transferred from the University of Pittsburgh's School of Public Health Library to the main University Archives, had not been thoroughly organized and indexed when I examined them, a situation that impaired more precise bibliographic citation. The transfer is now complete and an index available. Most of these papers relate to Parran's tenure as Surgeon General, although a number of files shed light on events in the early 1930s, and a collection of scrapbooks containing newspaper clippings was helpful in gaining a perspective on the media's perception of events in many different cities.

The records of the Public Health Service in the National Archives provided a wealth of information. For insight into the Service's strategy on the Parker bill, the four notebooks entitled *Records Regarding Coordination of Federal Public Health Activities, 1926–1929*, were a veritable gold mine. Also valuable were the General Subject Files and the General Records of the National Institute of Health. The latter contain some records dating back to 1915. These documents are in Record Group 90 at the National Archives. The Records of the Bureau of the Budget, housed in Record Group 51, were also enlightening about the Coolidge administration's point of view toward biomedical research. Many archivists, especially those in the Judicial, Fiscal, and Social Branch, cheerfully offered assistance in locating material even at a time when their staff had been severely reduced.

For a wide variety of primary and secondary sources, the collections of the National Library of Medicine proved invaluable. One cannot begin any study in medical history without consulting this library's *Bibliography of the History of Medicine*. In addition, the Division of the History of Medicine holds a number of manuscript collections that were useful, including oral histories, some documents pertaining to the early history of the Institute, unpublished manuscripts—especially those of Wyndham Miles relating to NIH and Public Health Service history—and an annotated manuscript and working notebooks for Bess Furman's *A Profile of the Public Health Service*. John B. Blake, director at that time, and his staff in the Division of the History of Medicine, especially Curator of Manuscripts Manfred Waserman, were always helpful in answering my multitude of questions.

Several divisions of the National Institutes of Health also allowed me access to information they had collected. Notable among these were the Office of Special Projects, under the direction of William Carrigan, who made available an oral history interview with W. Henry Sebrell prepared by that office. As a result of subsequent conversations and correspondence with Dr. Sebrell, that document will be transferred to the Sebrell Papers in the National Library of Medicine. Carrigan and Robert L. Schreiber of the Office of Communications, moreover, gave me access to a number of in-house documents relating to more recent research sponsored by the Institutes. J. Paul Van Nevel, director of the Office of Cancer Communications, allowed me to inspect the history files of the National Cancer Institute. Internal publications of the National Institutes of Health, such as the annual *NIH Almanac*, provided summarized information for reference.

A number of people at NIH kindly read and offered helpful comments on the epilogue to this book dealing with the more recent history of the Institutes. In addition to Carrigan, already mentioned, these people included Storm Whaley and Thomas Flavin of the Office of Communications, and Senior Scientific Advisor to the Director DeWitt Stetten, who also directed me to a number of sources and offered encouragement from the outset of this project.

For information on the political and scientific development of the Hygienic Laboratory and the National Institute of Health, the *Annual Reports* of the Public Health Service and its predecessors, the Public Health and Marine Hospital Service and the Marine Hospital Service, contained a wealth of information. These documents, although available elsewhere, were conveniently located in open stacks in the National Institutes of Health Library, which also had a variety of other useful documents pertaining to Service history. Among these were relevant congressional hearings; *Official List of Commissioned and Other Officers, 1897–1933*; various editions of *Regulations for the Government of the United States Public Health Service*; and a complete set of the *Public Health Reports* and *Bulletins of the Hygienic Laboratory*. Other publications by and about Service personnel also proved helpful and are well represented in the notes.

Interviews provide a source second to none for a personal perspective on events of any period. I was fortunate in being able to contact the only two surviving scientists from the Hygienic Laboratory, Sanford M. Rosenthal and W. Henry Sebrell. Dr. Rosenthal provided much information on the development of medicine and pharmacology in the early twentieth century and on the internal relationships of Service personnel in the late twenties. Dr. Sebrell's oral history also gave insights into the research work of the Hygienic Laboratory and the personnel involved. A. Baird Hastings, who was associated with the World War I fatigue studies of the Service and is now professor of chemistry at the University of California, San Diego, pointed out to me many of the developments in biochemistry that had a major effect on biomedical research. Michael B. Shimkin, former editor of the *Journal of the National Cancer Institute* and currently professor of community medicine at the University of California, San Diego, provided information from his encyclopedic memory on the 1930s that was especially valuable. I am indebted to all of these men for their kind cooperation.

For a nonscientist, the world of the laboratory can be bewildering. In attempting to understand the kinds of research procedures and instruments that were used in the 1920s, I found much information in the artifacts and trade catalogs available in the Medical Sciences Division, the National Museum of American History. A number of people in that division were always willing to entertain my questions and direct me to sources within the museum, including Curator Ramunas Kondratas, who was my advisor during my fellowship year at the museum, Curator Audrey Davis, and the late Everett Jackson, museum specialist.

The subject of private-sector funding for medical research was a knotty one. The very fact that money available for research was often not broken out separately in budgets revealed the minor role that research played in the early twentieth century. I relied heavily on two sources to make some judgment about this. Selma J. Mushkin, *Biomedical Research: Costs and Benefits* (Cambridge, Mass.: Ballinger Publishing Co., 1979), is the most recent work, although many amounts given were based on extrapolations from more recent data. The three *Bulletins of the National Research Council* on private-sector funding for research prepared in 1920, 1928, and 1934 and cited in chapter five were the only contemporary information available on the subject. For additional statistical information, *Historical Statistics of the United States*, prepared by the Bureau of the Census of the Department of Commerce, served as a standard reference.

A number of professional journals, newspapers, and popular magazines were rewarding sources of information and editorial opinion. The *Journal of the American Public Health Association* and the *Journal of the American Medical Association* were particularly useful in ascertaining the views of those organizations on increased federal funding for biomedical research. The *Journal of Industrial and Engineering Chemistry* under Charles Holmes Herty's editorship served as an effective mouthpiece for his point of view, but it also provided insight into the broader-ranging attitudes of professional chemists at that time. *Science*, the official organ of the American Association for the Advancement of Science, reflected the attitudes of the scientific community during World War I and the 1920s and continues to address the subject of federal support for science. For interpretative articles on scientific and medical history I have relied on a number of sources. In addition to the *Bibliography of the History of Medicine*, the annual "Critical Bibliography" in *Isis* provided excellent bibliographic assistance. The *Bulletin of the History of Medicine* and the *Journal of the History of Medicine and Allied Sciences* were indispensable sources. I also frequently consulted the *Journal of American History* and the *American Historical Review* for interpretative articles on the early twentieth century.

The *New York Times*, with its published indexes, was useful for news, editorial comment, and obituaries. Also helpful were articles in the *Washington Post*, the *Washington Star*, and several other newspapers. The *NIH Record*, an in-house publication, and *Public Affairs*, the newsletter of the Federation of American Societies for Experimental Biology, provided many articles of historical interest and current debate on federal funding for research. Popular magazines such as *Popular Science, Scientific American, Hygeia, Nation's Health, McClure's,* and *Good Housekeeping* chronicled the popular perception of medical research.

As this project progressed, I had many conversations with people who gave me factual information or interpretative ideas. Especially helpful were conversations with the late Robert L. Gordon, special assistant to the director of the National Institutes of Health; Merton England, historian for the National Science Foundation, to whom I am indebted also for a copy of his manuscript, now published, on the history of that organization; Marilyn Brachman Hoffman, Washington, D.C., who read the final chapter and directed me to several helpful sources during the course of the project; Nathan O. Kaplan, professor of chemistry at the University of California, San Diego; Michael J. Lacey of the Woodrow Wilson International Center for Scholars; Nathan Reingold, editor of the Joseph Henry Papers at the Smithsonian Institution; Nancy Knight, Brian Horrigan, Patricia Cooper, and G. Terry Sharrer at the National Museum of American History; and Caroline Hannaway and Jane Sewell at the Institute of the History of Medicine of the Johns Hopkins University Medical School. Although I never met some other people, I corresponded with them to my good advantage. P. Thomas Carroll and Jeffrey Sturchio were especially helpful in supplying information on the Chemical Foundation and on the development of chemistry as a profession in the early twentieth century. Barry D. Karl, professor of history at the University of Chicago, shared information on funding for research in the early twentieth century.

Three secondary sources were indispensable in approaching the history of the Public Health Service. These are Ralph C. Williams, *A History of the Public Health Service, 1798–1950* (Washington, D.C.: Commissioned Officers Association of the United States Public Health Service, 1951); Bess Furman, *A Profile of the United States Public Health Service, 1798–1948* (Washington, D.C.: Government Printing Office, DHEW Publication No. (NIH) 73-369); and Laurence F. Schmeckbier, *The Public Health Service: Its History, Activities, and Organization* (Baltimore: Johns Hopkins Press, 1923).

Richard Shryock's *American Medical Research Past and Present* (New York: Commonwealth Fund, 1947; reprint ed., New York: Arno Press, 1980) remains the best reference for an overall view of the trends in medical research in this country to World War II. Another of Shryock's books, *The Development of Modern Medicine: An Interpretation of the Social and Scientific Factors Involved* (New York: Alfred A. Knopf, 1936; reprint ed., Madison: University of Wisconsin Press, 1974), also provides a seminal interpretation of the social context in which scientific medicine began and flourished. A. Hunter Dupree's *Science in the Federal Government: A History of Policies and Activities to 1940* (Cambridge, Mass.: Belknap Press of Harvard University Press, 1957) was essential in placing medical research in the larger context of the federal science establishment. George Rosen's *A History of Public Health* (New York: MD Publications, 1958) and *Preventive Medicine in the United States, 1900–1975* (New York: Prodist, 1977) were fundamental reference works in public health. Derek J. deSolla Price's *Little Science, Big Science* (New York: Columbia University Press, 1963) was also crucial in conveying an understanding of how the scientific community grew in the early twentieth century.

Many secondary sources deal with the larger framework in which the story of the creation of the National Institute of Health was set. Key journal articles are referenced in the notes. Some of the most valuable books dealing with the history of medical research, public health, chemistry, pharmacy, and the broader setting in which these events occurred are: Erwin H. Ackerknecht,

A Short History of Medicine, rev. ed. (Baltimore: Johns Hopkins University Press, 1982); James Truslow Adams, *Our Business Civilization: Some Aspects of American Culture* (New York: Albert & Charles Boni, 1929); American Institute of the History of Pharmacy, *The Early Years of Federal Food and Drug Control* (Madison, Wis.: American Institute of the History of Pharmacy, 1982); Joseph Ben-David, *The Scientist's Role in Society* (Englewood Cliffs, N.J.: Prentice Hall, 1971); J. D. Bernal, *The Social Function of Science* (London: George Routledge & Sons, 1939); Thomas Neville Bonner, *American Doctors and German Universities: A Chapter in International Relations, 1870–1914* (Lincoln: University of Nebraska Press, 1963); John Z. Bowers and Elizabeth F. Purcell, eds., *Advances in American Medicine: Essays at the Bicentennial,* 2 vols. (New York: Josiah Macy, Jr., Foundation, 1976); John C. Burnham, ed., *Science in America: Historical Selections* (New York: Holt, Rinehart & Winston, 1971); James G. Burrow, *AMA: Voice of American Medicine* (Baltimore: Johns Hopkins Press, 1963); Burrow, *Organized Medicine in the Progressive Era: The Move toward Monopoly* (Baltimore: Johns Hopkins Press, 1977); Paul F. Clark, *Pioneer Microbiologists of America* (Madison: University of Wisconsin Press, 1961); George W. Corner, *A History of the Rockefeller Institute, 1901–1953: Origins and Growth* (New York: Rockefeller Institute Press, 1964); Harry F. Dowling, *Fighting Infection: Conquests of the Twentieth Century* (Cambridge, Mass.: Harvard University Press, 1977); John Duffy, *The Healers: A History of American Medicine* (Urbana: University of Illinois Press, 1976); A. Hunter Dupree, ed., *Science and the Emergence of Modern America, 1865–1916* (Chicago: Rand McNally & Co., 1963); Elizabeth W. Etheridge, *The Butterfly Caste: A Social History of Pellagra in the South* (Westport, Conn: Greenwood Publishing Co., 1972); Eduard Farber, *The Evolution of Chemistry: A History of Its Ideas, Methods, and Materials,* 2nd ed. (New York: Ronald Press Co., 1969); Morris Fishbein, *A History of the American Medical Association, 1847–1947* (Philadelphia: W. B. Saunders Co., 1947); Irving Fisher, *Report on National Vitality, Its Wastes and Conservation* (Washington, D.C.: Government Printing Office, 1923); Abraham Flexner, *Medical Education in the United States and Canada* (New York: Carnegie Foundation, 1910); Marcel Florkin, *A History of Biochemistry,* 4 vols. (Amsterdam and New York: Elsevier Scientific Publishing Co., 1972); Fielding H. Garrison, *An Introduction to the History of Medicine,* 4th ed. (Philadelphia: W. B. Saunders Co., 1929); Thomas H. Grainger, Jr., *A Guide to the History of Bacteriology* (New York: Ronald Press Co., 1958); A. McGehee Harvey, *Science at the Bedside: Clinical Research in American Medicine, 1905–1945* (Baltimore: Johns Hopkins University Press, 1981); Ellis W. Hawley, *The Great War and the Search for a Modern Order: A History of the American People and Their Institutions, 1917–1933* (New York: St. Martin's Press, 1979); Charles Holmes Herty et al., *The Future Independence and Progress of American Medicine in the Age of Chemistry* (New York: Chemical Foundation, 1921); Richard Hofstadter, *The Age of Reform: From Bryan to F.D.R.* (New York: Vintage Books, 1955); Aaron Ihde, *The Development of Modern Chemistry* (New York: Harper & Row, 1964); William Williams Keen, *Medical Research and Human Welfare* (Boston: Houghton Mifflin Co., 1917); Lester

S. King, ed., *Mainstreams of Medicine: Essays on the Social and Intellectual Context of Medical Practice* (Austin: University of Texas Press, 1971); Robert E. Kohler, *From Medical Chemistry to Biochemistry: The Making of a Biomedical Discipline* (Cambridge: Cambridge University Press, 1982); Victor H. Kramer, *The National Institute of Health: A Study in Public Administration* (New Haven: Quinnipiack Press, 1937); Adras P. Laborde, *A National Southerner: Ransdell of Louisiana* (New York: Benziger, 1951); Judith Walzer Leavitt and Ronald L. Numbers, eds., *Sickness and Health in America: Readings in the History of Medicine and Public Health* (Madison: University of Wisconsin Press, 1978); Robert D. Leigh, *Federal Health Administration in the United States* (New York: Harper & Bros., 1927); Jacques Loeb, *The Mechanistic Conception of Life* (Chicago: University of Chicago Press, 1912); Robert S. Lynd and Helen M. Lynd, *Middletown: A Study in Contemporary American Culture* (New York: Harcourt, Brace & Co., 1929); Elmer Verner McCollum, *A History of Nutrition: The Sequence of Ideas in Nutrition Investigations* (Boston: Houghton Mifflin Co., 1957); Donald R. McCoy, *Calvin Coolidge: The Quiet President* (New York: MacMillan Co., 1969); Thomas McKeown, *The Modern Rise of Population* (London: Edward Arnold, 1976); Harry H. Moore, *Public Health in the United States* (New York: Harper & Bros., 1923); Robert K. Murray, *The Politics of Normalcy: Governmental Theory and Practice in the Harding-Coolidge Era* (New York: W. W. Norton & Co., 1973); Joseph Needham, ed., *The Chemistry of Life: Eight Lectures on the History of Biochemistry* (Cambridge: Cambridge University Press, 1971); Arthur Newsholme, *Evolution of Preventive Medicine* (Baltimore: Williams & Wilkins Co., 1927); Ronald L. Numbers, *Almost Persuaded: American Physicians and Compulsory Health Insurance, 1912–1920* (Baltimore: Johns Hopkins University Press, 1978); William Osler, *The Evolution of Modern Medicine* (New Haven: Yale University Press, 1922); John Parascandola, ed., *The History of Antibiotics: A Symposium* (Madison: American Institute of the History of Pharmacy, 1980); John Parascandola and James Whorton, eds., *Chemistry and Modern Society: Historical Essays in Honor of Aaron J. Ihde* (Washington, D.C.: American Chemical Society, 1983); President's Research Committee on Social Trends, *Recent Social Trends in the United States*, 2 vols. (New York: McGraw-Hill Book Co., 1933); Don Krasher Price, *Government and Science: Their Dynamic Relation in American Democracy* (New York: New York University Press, 1954); Price, *The Scientific Estate* (Cambridge, Mass.: Belknap Press of Harvard University Press, 1967); Nathan Reingold, ed., *The Sciences in the American Context: New Perspectives* (Washington, D.C.: Smithsonian Institution Press, 1979); Nathan Reingold and Ida H. Reingold, eds., *Science in America: A Documentary History, 1900–1939* (Chicago: University of Chicago Press, 1981); Stanley Joel Reiser, *Medicine and the Reign of Technology* (Cambridge: Cambridge University Press, 1978); Charles E. Rosenberg, *No Other Gods: On Science and American Social Thought* (Baltimore: Johns Hopkins University Press, 1976); Karl E. Rothschuch, *History of Physiology*, trans. and ed. Guenter B. Risse (Huntington, N.Y.: Robert E. Krieger Publishing Co., 1973; original German edition, 1953); Richard H. Shryock, *National Tuberculosis Association, 1904–1954: A Study of the Vol-*

untary Health Movement in the United States (New York: National Tuberculosis Association, 1957); Henry E. Sigerst, *On the Sociology of Medicine* (New York: MD Publications, 1960); Preston William Slosson, *The Great Crusade and After, 1914–1928* (New York: Macmillan Co., 1930); Wilson G. Smillie, *Public Health Administration in the United States* (New York: Macmillan Co., 1936); Smillie, *Public Health: Its Promise for the Future* (New York: Macmillan Co., 1955); Paul Starr, *The Social Transformation of American Medicine* (New York: Basic Books, 1983); Rosemary Stevens, *American Medicine and the Public Interest* (New Haven: Yale University Press, 1971); Julius Stieglitz, ed., *Chemistry in Medicine* (New York: Chemical Foundation, 1928); Stephen P. Strickland, *Politics, Science, and Dread Disease: A Short History of United States Medical Research Policy* (Cambridge, Mass.: Harvard University Press, 1972); Lloyd C. Taylor, Jr., *The Medical Profession and Social Reform, 1885–1945* (New York: St. Martin's Press, 1974); Milton Terris, ed., *Goldberger on Pellagra* (Baton Rouge: Louisiana State University Press, 1964); James A. Tobey, *The National Government and Public Health* (Baltimore: Johns Hopkins Press, 1926); Ronald C. Tobey, *The American Ideology of National Science, 1919–1930* (Pittsburgh: University of Pittsburgh Press, 1971); U.S., National Resources Committee, Science Committee, *Research—A National Resource*, 3 vols. (Washington, D.C.: Government Printing Office, 1938–41); U.S., National Resources Committee, Science Committee, *Technological Trends and National Policy, Including the Social Implication of New Inventions* (Washtingotn, D.C.: Government Printing Office, 1937); Robert H. Wiebe, *The Search for Order, 1877–1920* (New York: Hill & Wang, 1967); Charles-Edward Armory Winslow, *The Evoloution and Significance of the Modern Public Health Campaign* (New Haven: Yale University Press, 1923); James Harvey Young, *The Medical Messiahs: A Social History of Health Quackery in the Twentieth Century* (Princeton: Princeton University Press, 1967); Young, *The Toadstool Millionaires: A Social History of Patent Medicines in America before Federal Regulation* (Princeton: Princeton University Press, 1961).

Notes

Introduction: Inventing the NIH

1. Office of Program Planning and Evaluation, *NIH Data Book*, 1983 (Washington, D.C.: U.S. Department of Health and Human Services, National Institutes of Health, 1983), pp. 4, 51.

2. Selected examples of this debate include C. W. Sherwin and R. S. Isenson, *First Interim Report on Project Hindsight* (Washington, D.C.: Office of Director of Defense Research and Engineering, June 30, 1966); James A. Shannon, "NIH—Present and Potential Contribution to Application of Biomedical Knowledge," in *Research in the Service of Man: Biomedical Knowledge, Development, and Use,* U.S. Senate Doc. 55, 90th Cong., 1st sess., 1967, pp. 72–85; M. B. Visscher, "Applied Science and Medical Progress," in *Applied Science and Technological Progress* (Washington, D.C.: National Academy of Sciences, 1967), pp. 185–206; J. H. Comroe and R. D. Dripps, "Scientific Basis for the Support of Biomedical Sciences," *Science* 192: 105–11 (April 9, 1976).

3. "How Much for Science?" *Washington Post,* February 3, 1982, p. A22.

4. Robert M. Bock to Henry A. Waxman, March 13, 1980, in the Federation of American Societies for Experimental Biology newsletter, *Public Affairs* 39(5): ii (April 1980).

5. For what is still the best overall survey of the activities of the federal government in science, see A. Hunter Dupree, *Science in the Federal Government: A History of Policies and Activities to 1940* (Cambridge, Mass.: Belknap Press of Harvard University Press, 1957).

6. A. Hunter Dupree, "Central Scientific Organization in the United States Government," *Minerva* 1: 453–69 (Summer 1963).

7. This argument is the subject of Barry Dean Karl's essay "Philanthropy, Policy Planning, and the Bureaucratization of the Democratic Ideal," *Daedalus* 129–49 (Fall 1976).

8. Atherton Seidell, "The Berthelot Centenary and the Resulting International Efforts to Advance Chemistry" (Address before the joint meeting of chemical societies at the Chemists' Club, New York, April 6, 1928), *Science* 67: 498 (May 18, 1928). An expanded analysis of this orientation in American thought is in J.G.A. Pocock, "Civic Humanism and Its Role in Anglo-American Thought," in his *Politics, Language, and Time: Essays on Political Thought and History* (New York: Atheneum Publishers, 1971), pp. 80–103.

9. George Rosen, "Critical Levels in the Historical Process: A Theoretical Exploration Dedicated to Henry Ernest Sigerist," *Journal of the History of Medicine and Allied Sciences* 13: 179–85 (April 1958); hereafter cited as *JHMAS*.

One: A Laboratory of Hygiene

1. U.S. Treasury Department, Marine Hospital Service, *Annual Report of the Supervising Surgeon of the Marine Hospital Service of the United States* (Washington, D.C.: 1888), p. 11. Hereafter cited as MHS *Annual Report* for indicated year.

2. Phyllis Allen Richmond, "American Attitudes toward the Germ Theory of Disease (1860–1880)," in Gert H. Brieger, ed., *Theory and Practice in American Medicine: Historical Studies from the Journal of the History of Medicine and Allied Sciences* (New York: Science History Publications, 1976), pp. 58–84. This article was first published in *JHMAS* 9: 428–54 (1954).

3. The European research institutes are discussed in John B. Blake, "Scientific Institutions since the Renaissance: Their Role in Medical Research," *Proceedings of the American Philosophical Society* 101: 31–62 (February 15, 1957).

4. C.-E.A. Winslow, "The Laboratory in the Service of the State," *American Journal of Public Health* 6: 222–33 (1915); reprinted in *Health Laboratory Science* 9:5–15 (January 1972). Hereafter the *American Journal of Public Health* is cited as *AJPH*. In 1928 the *Journal* merged with *Nation's Health*. References to these combined publications are also cited as *AJPH*.

5. See, for example, Charles Rosenberg, *The Cholera Years* (Chicago: University of Chicago Press, 1962), especially pp. 82–98.

6. On the establishment of the Marine Hospital Service see Ralph C. Williams, *The United States Public Health Service, 1798–1950* (Washington, D.C.: Commissioned Officers Association of the United States Public Health Service, 1951), pp. 23–46. Hereafter cited as Williams, *USPHS*.

7. George Rosen, *A History of Public Health*, MD Monographs on Medical History, no. 1 (New York: MD Publications, 1958), pp. 233–50.

8. For biographical information on Billings see Fielding H. Garrison, *John Shaw Billings: A Memoir,* (New York: G. P. Putnam's Sons, 1915); Frank Bradway Rogers, "John Shaw Billings: 1838–1913," *Library Journal* 88: 2622–24 (July 1963).

9. *An Act to Reorganize the Marine Hospital Service, and to Provide for the Relief of Sick and Disabled Seamen,* June 29, 1870, ch. 169, 16 *Stat. L.* 169.

10. Bess Furman, *A Profile of the United States Public Health Service, 1798–1948* (Washington, D.C.: Government Printing Office, DHEW Publication No. (NIH) 73-369), pp. 109, 114–23. Hereafter cited as Furman, *Profile.* For biographical information on Woodworth, see Williams, *USPHS,* pp. 472–75.

11. Christopher C. Cox, "A Report upon the Necessity of a National Sanitary Bureau," in *Public Health; Reports and Papers Presented at the Meetings of the American Public Health Association in the Year 1873,* vol. 1 (New York: American Public Health Association, 1875), pp. 522–32, as cited in R. D. Leigh, *Federal Health Administration in the United States* (New York: Harper & Bros., 1927), pp. 464 and 614, note 1. A summary of the activities of the first fifty years of the American Public Health Association is in Mazyck P. Ravenel, ed., *A Half Century of Public Health,* Jubilee Historical Volume (New York: American Public Health Association, 1921).

12. Henry I. Bowditch, "The Future Health Council of the Nation," *Transactions of the American Medical Association* 26: 301–14 (1875).

13. For detailed studies of the National Board of Health see Peter Bruton, "The National Board of Health" (Ph.D. dissertation, University of Maryland, 1974); Wyndham D. Miles, "A History of the National Board of Health, 1879–1893," 2 vols., unpublished manuscript, National Library of Medicine, 1970.

14. Furman, *Profile,* pp. 148–49. For biographical information on Hamilton see Williams, *USPHS,* pp. 475–77; Howard A. Kelly, *A Cyclopedia of American Medical Biography: Comprising the Lives of Eminent Deceased Physicians and Surgeons from 1610 to 1910,* 2 vols. (Philadelphia: W. B. Saunders Co., 1912), 1: 379. Although Hamilton served as editor of the *Journal of the American Medical Association* for five years, neither the *Journal* nor histories of the association contain significant biographical information about him.

15. U.S. Treasury Department, Marine Hospital Service, *Report of the Supervising Surgeon General on the Arguments before the Committee on Commerce of the House of Representatives, concerning the Proposed Establishment of a Bureau of Health,* Treasury Department Doc. 1092 (Washington, D.C.: Government Printing Office, 1888).

16. MHS *Annual Report,* 1888, p. 11.

17. Williams, *USPHS,* p. 473; Furman, *Profile,* p. 123.

18. For biographical information on Wyman see his obituary in the *Journal of the American Medical Association* 57: 1778 (November 25, 1911); Williams, *USPHS,* pp. 477–79; Furman, *Profile,* pp. 199–201. Hereafter the *Journal of the American Medical Association* is cited as *JAMA.*

19. For biographical information on Kinyoun see Paul F. Clark, *Pioneer Microbiologists of America* (Madison: University of Wisconsin Press, 1961), pp. 206–7; Williams, *USPHS,* pp. 249–50; Furman, *Profile,* pp. 202–3; J. McKeen Cattell, ed., *American Men of Science,* 2nd ed. (New York: Science Press, 1910), pp. 260–61.

20. MHS *Annual Report,* 1888, p. 11. No one has been able to state

absolutely which room in the structure housed the laboratory. It may have been an attic room destroyed in later remodeling.

21. Ibid.

22. Ibid.

23. "The Research Program of the U.S. Public Health Service," *AJPH* 42: 995–96 (August 1952).

24. MHS *Annual Report,* 1888, p. 11.

25. In 1890 and 1893 the Service received new power over interstate quarantine and additional powers over maritime quarantine. In 1890 it was also charged with the medical inspection of immigrants. See U.S. Treasury Department, "Laws Relating to the Public Health Service," *United States Public Health Service Regulations* (Washington, D.C.: Government Printing Office, 1931), pp. 179–95.

26. Arthur M. Stimson, "A Brief History of Bacteriological Investigations of the United States Public Health Service," *Public Health Reports,* Supplement 141 (1938), p. 5. Hereafter cited as Stimson, "Bacteriological Investigations."

27. MHS *Annual Report,* 1895, p. 311.

28. Ibid., p. 334.

29. Ibid., p. 327.

30. An expanded discussion of this legislation is in ch. 2.

31. MHS *Annual Report,* 1891, p. 10.

32. MHS *Annual Report,* 1895, pp. 329, 340. One of the first bottles of diphtheria antitoxin produced at the Hygienic Laboratory is in the collection of the Medical Sciences Division, National Museum of American History, Smithsonian Institution, Washington, D.C.

33. MHS *Annual Report,* 1894, p. 188.

34. Stimson, "Bacteriological Investigations," p. 65.

35. U.S. Congress, House Committee on Ventilation and Acoustics, *Ventilation of the House of Representatives,* House Rept. 853, 53rd Cong., 2nd sess., May 8, 1894, as quoted in Furman, *Profile,* pp. 213–14.

36. MHS *Annual Report,* 1894, p. 189.

37. Ibid., 1900, p. 670.

38. U.S. Treasury Department, Public Health Service, *Annual Report of the Surgeon General of the Public Health Service of the United States* (Washington, D.C.: Government Printing Office, 1914), p. 83; 1915, p. 82. Hereafter cited as PHS *Annual Report* for indicated year.

39. PHS *Annual Report,* 1922, p. 66. Because of the disruptions of World War I, the school was discontinued from 1918 until 1922.

40. For an account of Kinyoun's departure from the laboratory and involvement with the San Francisco plague epidemic, see Furman, *Profile,* pp. 220–21; 244–48; quotation is from p. 248.

41. Clark, *Pioneer Microbiologists,* pp. 206–7.

42. Kinyoun was relieved from duty as director in April 1899. E. K. Sprague was appointed acting director until Rosenau assumed the post of director on October 25, 1899. For biographical information on Rosenau see George Ro-

sen's sketch of him in Edward T. James and John A. Garraty, eds., *Dictionary of American Biography* (New York: Charles Scribner's Sons, 1928–80), supplement 4 (1974), pp. 700–2; L. D. Felton, "Milton J. Rosenau, 1869–1946," *Journal of Bacteriology* 53: 1–3 (1947); and Williams, *USPHS*, pp. 250–51.

43. On typhoid fever in the Spanish American War and the public health measures used to control it see Martha L. Sternberg, *George Miller Sternberg: A Biography* (Chicago: American Medical Association, 1920), p. 185; Walter Reed, Victor C. Vaughan, and Edward O. Shakespeare, *Report on the Origin and Spread of Typhoid Fever in U.S. Military Camps during the Spanish War of 1898* (Washington, D.C.: Government Printing Office, 1904).

44. MHS *Annual Report*, 1898, p. 828.

45. Leigh, *Federal Health Administration*, p. 484.

46. MHS *Annual Report*, 1899, p. 861.

47. Ibid., 1901, p. 592.

48. U.S. Congress, House Committee on Interstate and Foreign Commerce, *Hearings before the Committee on Interstate and Foreign Commerce on Bills Relating to Health Activities of the General Government*, 61st Cong., 2nd sess., and 61st Cong., 3rd sess., June 1910 and January 1911 (printed as one volume entitled *Health Activities of the General Government, Hearings, 61st Congress, 1910–1911*), p. 621. Hereafter cited as *Health Activities Hearings, 1910–1911*.

49. *Sundry Civil Appropriation Act*, March 3, 1901, ch. 863, 31 *Stat. L.* 1137. March 3, 1901, was a day for advancing science in the federal government. Congress also created the National Bureau of Standards on that day. See Daniel J. Kevles, *The Physicists: The History of a Scientific Community in Modern America* (New York: Alfred A. Knopf, 1978), pp. 66–67.

50. Dupree, *Science in the Federal Government*, pp. 216–17.

51. *Health Activities Hearings, 1910–1911*, p. 621.

52. Ibid.

53. *An Act to Increase the Efficiency and Change the Name of the United States Marine Hospital Service*, July 1, 1902, ch. 1370, 32 *Stat. L.* 712.

54. U.S. Congress, Senate Committee on Public Health and National Quarantine, *Relative to the Marine-Hospital Service, Etc.*, Senate Rept. 1531 to Accompany S. 2162, 57th Cong., 1st sess., May 14, 1902, p. 1.

55. Ibid., p. 2.

56. Ibid., p. 3.

57. U.S. Treasury Department, Public Health and Marine Hospital Service, *Annual Report of the Surgeon General of the United States Public Health and Marine Hospital Service* (Washington, D.C.: Government Printing Office, 1906), p. 232. Hereafter cited as PH-MHS *Annual Report* for indicated year.

58. Ibid., 1908, p. 83.

59. Stimson, "Bacteriological Investigations," p. 65; the results of the investigation were published in the *Bulletin of the Hygienic Laboratory* 35 (1907), 44 (1907), 52 (1909), 78 (1911), entire issues. Hereafter cited as *BHL*.

60. Stimson, "Bacteriological Investigations," p. 66.

61. U.S. Congress, Senate Committee on Public Health and National Quarantine, *Relative to the Marine-Hospital Service, Etc.*, Senate Rept. 1531 to Accompany S. 2162, 57th Cong., 1st sess., May 14, 1902, p. 2.

62. *An Act to Regulate Appointments in the Marine Hospital Service of the United States*, January 4, 1889, ch. 19, 25 *Stat. L.* 639; Williams, *USPHS*, pp. 490–92.

63. PH-MHS *Annual Report*, 1902, p. 44.

64. Ibid., 1906, p. 227; 1907, p. 45; 1909, p. 79; PHS *Annual Report*, 1918, pp. 59–60.

65. PH-MHS *Annual Report*, 1903, p. 326.

66. MHS *Annual Report*, 1900, p. 682; U.S. Congress, *Joint Resolution Providing for the Publication of the Annual Reports and Bulletins of the Hygienic Laboratory and of the Yellow Fever Institute of the Public Health and Marine Hospital Service*, Joint Resolution No. 21, February 24, 1905, 33 *Stat. L.* 1283; for a list of the *Bulletins* published before January 1927 see U.S. Treasury Department, Public Health Service, *Publications of the United States Public Health Service*, Miscellaneous Publication No. 12 (Washington, D.C.: Government Printing Office, 1927), pp. 22–30.

67. For biographical information on Anderson, see Williams, *USPHS*, pp. 251–52; and Clark, *Pioneer Microbiologists*, p. 211. McCoy's biography is given in the discussion of his directorship in ch. 8.

68. For biographical information on Stiles see James H. Cassedy's sketch of him, "Charles Wardell Stiles," in Edward T. James, ed., *Dictionary of American Biography* (New York: Charles Scribner's Sons, 1928–80), supplement 3 (1973), pp. 737–39; John Ettling, *The Germ of Laziness: Rockefeller Philanthropy and Public Health in the New South* (Cambridge, Mass.: Harvard University Press, 1981), pp. 9–48; an autobiographical article by Stiles is "Early History, in Part Esoteric, of the Hookworm (Uncinariasis) Campaign in Our Southern U.S.," *Journal of Parasitology* 25: 283–308 (August 1939); obituaries in the *Journal of Parasitology* 27:195–201 (June 1941) and the *New York Times,* January 25, 1941; see also "Charles Wardell Stiles," in Jeanette Barry, comp., *Notable Contributions to Medical Research by Public Health Service Scientists: A Bibliography to 1940* (Washington, D.C.: U.S. Department of Health, Education & Welfare, Public Health Service, 1960), pp. 82–86. Hereafter cited as *Notable Contributions.*

69. Cassedy, "Charles Wardell Stiles," p. 738.

70. Ibid.

71. George Rosen, "The Bacteriological, Immunologic, and Chemotherapeutic Period—1875–1950," *Bulletin of the New York Academy of Medicine*, second series, 40: 483–94 (June 1964).

72. Stimson, "Bacteriological Investigations," table of contents listing, p. iii.

73. Williams, *USPHS*, p. 190; much of the research on tularemia was published in "Tularemia Francis, 1921," *BHL* 130 (1922), entire issue.

74. Alice C. Evans, "Further Studies on Bacterium Abortus and Related Bacteria. II. A Comparison of Bacterium Abortus with Bacterium Bronchi-

septicus and with the Organism which Causes Malta Fever," *Journal of Infectious Diseases* 22: 580–93 (1918); "Malta Fever; Cattle Suggested as a Possible Source of Infection, following a Serological Study of Humans," *Public Health Reports* 39: 501–18 (1924); "Studies on Brucella (Alkaligens) Melitensis," *BHL* 143 (1925), entire issue.

75. For a discussion of the development and contributions of biochemistry see Eduard Farber, *The Evolution of Chemistry: A History of Its Ideas, Methods, and Materials,* 2nd ed. (New York: Ronald Press Co., 1969), ch. 23; Robert E. Kohler, *From Medical Chemistry to Biochemistry: The Making of a Biomedical Discipline* (Cambridge: Cambridge University Press, 1982); Marcel Florkin, *A History of Biochemistry,* 4 vols. (Amsterdam: Elsevier, 1972–79); A. McGehee Harvey, *Science at the Bedside: Clinical Research in American Medicine, 1905–1945* (Baltimore: Johns Hopkins University Press, 1981), especially p. 47.

76. For an overview of physiological research in the twentieth century see Karl E. Rothschuh, *History of Physiology,* trans. and ed. Guenter B. Risse (Huntington, N.Y: Robert E. Krieger Publishing Co., 1973), pp. 264–368; on bacteriological research see E. F. Gale, "The Development of Microbiology," in Joseph Needham, ed., *The Chemistry of Life: Eight Lectures on the History of Biochemistry* (Cambridge: Cambridge University Press, 1971), pp. 38–59.

77. On the history of vitamin research see Elmer V. McCollum, *A History of Nutrition: The Sequence of Ideas in Nutrition Investigations* (Boston: Houghton Mifflin Co., 1957).

78. For biographical information on Kastle see *Notable Contributions,* pp. 48–49; Wyndham Miles, "Joseph Hoeing Kastle," in Miles, ed., *American Chemists and Chemical Engineers* (Washington, D.C.: American Chemical Society, 1976), pp. 262–63. Kastle assumed the division directorship June 26, 1905.

79. Kastle's work on oxidases was published in *BHL* 26 (1906); 31 (1906); and 59 (1909), entire issues. His new reagent for determining hydrochloric acid in gastric contents was published in the *Journal of Biological Chemistry* 3: xi–xii (1907).

80. PH-MHS *Annual Report,* 1907, p. 57. Kastle's work on blood was published in *BHL* 51 (1909).

81. For a discussion of the history of such studies see Abraham M. Lilienfeld, *"Ceteris Paribus:* The Evolution of the Clinical Trial," *Bulletin of the History of Medicine* 56: 1–18 (Spring 1982). Hereafter, the *Bulletin of the History of Medicine* is cited as *BHM.* James H. Cassedy, in *American Medicine and Statistical Thinking, 1800–1860* (Cambridge, Mass.: Harvard University Press, 1984), discusses early attempts to evaluate the efficacy of drugs by statistical methods; see especially pp. 73, 75–77.

82. James Harvey Young, "Public Policy and Drug Innovation," *Pharmacy in History* 24: 3–7 (1982); M. L. Tainter and G.M.A. Marcelli, "The Rise of Synthetic Drugs in the American Pharmaceutical Industry," *Bulletin of the New York Academy of Medicine* 35: 402 (1959); Robert G. Denkewalter and

Max Tishler, "Drug Research—Whence and Wither," in E. Jucker, ed., *Fortschritte der Arzneimittelforschung*, vol. 10 (Basel and Stuttgart: Birkhauser, 1966), pp. 11–31.

83. Raymond F. Bacon, "The Value of Research to Industry," *Science* 40: 874–75 (December 18, 1914); see also the article by Carl Voegtlin, chief of the Division of Pharmacology of the Hygienic Laboratory, on advances in pharmacology, "The Hope of Mankind—Chemotherapy," in Julius Stieglitz, ed., *Chemistry in Medicine: A Cooperative Treatise Intended to Give Examples of Progress Made in Medicine with the Aid of Chemistry* (New York: Chemical Foundation, 1928), pp. 701–20; a historical account of these developments is in William N. Hubbard, Jr., "The Origins of Medicinals," in John Z. Bowers and Elizabeth F. Purcell, eds., *Advances in American Medicine: Essays at the Bicentennial*, 2 vols. (New York: Josiah Macy, Jr. Foundation, 1976), 2: 685–721.

84. For biographical information on Hunt see "Reid Hunt," in *Notable Contributions*, pp. 43–47; Otto Krayer, "Reid Hunt," in Edward T. James and John A. Garraty, eds., *Dictionary of American Biography* (New York: Charles Scribner's Sons, 1928–80), supplement 4 (1974), pp. 410–12; "Reid Hunt," *Harvard Medical Alumni Bulletin* 23: 39–42 (1949); E. K. Marshall, Jr., "Reid Hunt," *Biographical Memoirs* (National Academy of Sciences) 26: 25–44 (1951). Hunt was appointed chief of the division March 1, 1904.

85. Reid Hunt and R. de M. Taveau, "On the Physiological Action of Certain Cholin Derivatives and New Methods for Detecting Cholin," *British Medical Journal* 2: 1788–91 (1906).

86. *Notable Contributions*, p. 45. Hunt's work was published as "Studies in Experimental Alcoholism," *BHL* 33 (1907), entire issue.

87. Reid Hunt, "The Acetonitrile Test for Thyroid and Some Alterations of Metabolism," *American Journal of Physiology* 63: 257–99 (1923).

88. These awards are noted in *Notable Contributions*, pp. xi–xiv. Portions of this chart have been updated and reproduced in Appendix A.

89. Paul de Kruif, *The Hunger Fighters* (New York: Harcourt, Brace & Co., 1928); ch. 5, "The Automatic Man: Francis," relates the story of Edward Francis's work on tularemia; ch. 11, "The Soft-Spoken Desperado: Goldberger," tells of Joseph Goldberger's research on pellagra. *Men Against Death* (New York: Harcourt, Brace & Co., 1932); ch. 4, "Spencer: In the Happy Valley," discusses Roscoe Spencer's work on Rocky Mountain spotted fever; ch. 5, "Evans: Death in Milk," tells of Alice Evans's research on undulant fever; ch. 6, "McCoy: Should Generals Die in Bed?" relates the work of George McCoy on psittacosis.

90. *Health Activities Hearings, 1910–1911*, p. 626. The speaker was Dr. G. Lloyd Magruder.

91. PH-MHS *Annual Report*, 1911, p. 78.

92. A summary table of the research appropriations and staff for the years 1907 to 1936 is in Victoria A. Harden, "Toward a National Institute of Health: The Development of Federal Biomedical Research Policy, 1900–1930" (Ph.D. dissertation, Emory University, 1983), p. 143.

93. John W. Kerr, "Travels of a Sanitarian: Being the Experience of a

Lifetime in the U.S. Public Health Service, 1898–1934," unpublished manuscript in possession of his daughter, Helen Pratt Kerr Grismer.

Chapter Two: Institutionalization and Development in the Progressive Era

1. PH-MHS *Annual Report,* 1907, p. 15.
2. Upton B. Sinclair, *The Jungle* (New York: Vanguard, 1906); Samuel Hopkins Adams, *The Great American Fraud* (n.p.: Collier & Son, 1905–6); James H. Cassedy, "Muckraking and Medicine: Samuel Hopkins Adams," *American Quarterly* 16: 85–99 (1964).
3. For a discussion of the passage and initial enforcement of this act see Ramunas A. Kondratas, "Biologics Control Act of 1902," in *The Early Years of Federal Food and Drug Control* (Madison, Wis.: American Institute of the History of Pharmacy, 1982), pp. 8–27.
4. PH-MHS *Annual Report,* 1905, p. 221; 1908, p. 46; Kondratas, "Biologics Control Act of 1902," p. 20.
5. PH-MHS *Annual Report,* 1908, p. 43.
6. See the following PHS *Annual Reports:* 1917, p. 61; 1922, p. 66; 1924, pp. 54–55.
7. PH-MHS *Annual Report,* 1900, p. 669.
8. A list of firms licensed in 1908 is in the PH-MHS *Annual Report,* 1908, p. 44.
9. Milton J. Rosenau and John F. Anderson, "A Study of the Cause of Sudden Death Following the Injection of Horse Serum," *BHL* 29 (1906), entire issue.
10. John F. Anderson and W. H. Frost, "Studies upon Anaphylaxis with Special Reference to the Antibodies Concerned," *BHL* 64 (1910), entire issue.
11. Stimson, "Bacteriological Investigations," p. 49.
12. Ibid.
13. PH-MHS *Annual Report,* 1908, p. 56; PHS *Annual Report,* 1921, p. 85.
14. U.S. Congress, House Committee on Interstate and Foreign Commerce, *Hearings Before the Committee on Interstate and Foreign Commerce on Public Health and Marine Hospital Service,* No. 2, 60th Cong., 2nd sess., January 1909, p. 5.
15. For a discussion of pellagra in the South see Elizabeth W. Etheridge, *The Butterfly Caste: A Social History of Pellagra in the South* (Westport, Conn.: Greenwood Publishing Co., 1972). Goldberger's research was published in a variety of articles in the *Public Health Reports* and the Hygienic Laboratory *Bulletin,* some of which are assembled in Milton Terris, ed., *Goldberger on Pellagra* (Baton Rouge: Louisiana State University Press, 1964).
16. J. W. Kerr, "Scientific Research by the Public Health Service," *Annals of the American Academy of Political and Social Science* 37: 27 (March 1911).
17. U.S. Congress, House, *Congressional Record,* 61st Cong., 3rd sess., February 27, 1911, p. 3621.
18. The discrepancies between military and Service officers were discussed

at many hearings. See, for example, *Arguments in Favor of the Proposed Measure to Promote Efficiency of the United States Public Health and Marine Hospital Service (Personnel)*, presented to the Committee on Interstate and Foreign Commerce on bills pending in 1908; and U.S. Congress, House Committee on Interstate and Foreign Commerce, House Rept. 2000 to Accompany H.R. 18794, 60th Cong., 2nd sess., 1909. Both are reprinted in *Health Activities Hearings, 1910–1911*, pp. 501–12.

19. U.S. Congress, Senate Committee on Public Health and National Quarantine, *Relative to the Marine-Hospital Service, Etc.*, Senate Rept. 1531 to Accompany S. 2162, 57th Cong., 1st sess., May 14, 1902, p. 2.

20. C. W. Stiles, Reid Hunt, and Joseph Kastle to Walter Wyman, February 1, 1909, File 5017, United States Public Health Service General Subject Files, 1924–35, Records of the Public Health Service, Record Group 90, National Archives, Washington, D.C. Hereafter cited as PHS General Subject Files, 1924–35, PHS Records, RG 90, NA. In this letter of complaint, the three Professors reminded Wyman of the unfulfilled promises he had made.

21. Ibid.

22. Ibid.

23. Wyndham Miles, "Congress Broadens the PHS's Authority to Investigate Disease, 1912," unpublished manuscript, National Library of Medicine, n.d., p. 21.

24. In *Conservation and the Gospel of Efficiency: The Progressive Conservation Movement, 1890–1920* (Cambridge: Harvard University Press, 1959), Samuel P. Hays discussed the development of the conservation movement and its expansion into areas originally unforeseen, such as public health. See especially pp. 176–77.

25. Robert Wiebe elucidated this orientation of the Progressives in *The Search for Order, 1877–1920* (New York: Hill & Wang, 1967).

26. J. Pease Norton, "The Economic Advisability of Inaugurating a National Department of Health," *JAMA* 47: 1003–7 (1906); quotations are from pp. 1005, 1006.

27. On the Committee of One Hundred, see Manfred Waserman, "The Quest for a National Health Department in the Progressive Era," *BHM* 49: 353–80 (Fall 1975); George Rosen, "The Committee of One Hundred on National Health and the Campaign for a National Health Department, 1906–1912," *AJPH* 62: 261–63 (February 1972); W. J. Schieffelin, "Work of the Committee of One Hundred on National Health," *Annals of the American Academy of Political and Social Science* 37: 321–30 (March 1911).

28. This letter by J. Pease Norton was sent to Milton J. Rosenau, director of the Hygienic Laboratory. It is in the Rosenau Collection of the School of Public Health, University of North Carolina at Chapel Hill, and is cited in Rosen, "Committee of One Hundred," pp. 261–262. It is reprinted here by permission of Michel A. Ibrahim, Dean.

29. Irving Fisher, *Report on National Vitality: Its Wastes and Conservation*, Bulletin 30 of the Committee of One Hundred on National Health (Washington, D.C.: Government Printing Office, 1923), p. 126. The report was originally printed as S. Doc. 419, 61st Cong., 2nd sess. (1910).

30. Theodore Roosevelt, Seventh Annual Message, December 3, 1907, *Messages and Papers of the Presidents*, 20 vols. (New York: Bureau of National Literature, 1897–1927), 14: 7104; Eighth Annual Message, December 8, 1908, ibid., 14: 7229.

31. William Howard Taft, First Annual Message, December 7, 1909, ibid., 15: 7438.

32. *A Bill Establishing a Department of Public Health, and for Other Purposes*, S. 6049, 61st Cong., 2nd sess., February 1, 1910. A copy of the bill is in File 4689, Public Health Service General Subject Files, 1897–1923, Public Health Service Records, Record Group 90, National Archives. Hereafter cited as PHS General Subject Files, 1897–1923, PHS Records, RG 90, NA.

33. Irving Fisher to George Shiras, March 11, 1910; Fisher to William G. Eliot, Jr., March 11, 1910, in Irving Fisher Papers, Yale University Library, New Haven, Conn., as quoted in Waserman, "Quest for a National Health Department," p. 367, footnote 61.

34. Walter Wyman to President William Howard Taft, June 21, 1909, quoted in U.S. Congress, House, *Congressional Record*, 61st Cong., 2nd sess., March 24, 1910, p. 3649.

35. *Health Activities Hearings, 1910–1911*, p. 497.

36. Wyman's goals are presumed from the statement of Congressman Mann, who introduced H.R. 24875 (61st Cong., 2nd sess.) containing these measures. Referring to President Taft's recommendation that a bureau of health be established, Mann said, "I asked Doctor Wyman to prepare a bill which would give, in a way, his views upon this subject, and that is this bill H.R. 24875." See *Health Activities Hearings, 1910–1911*, p. 206. A copy of Mann's bill is in these hearings, pp. 12–14.

37. Copies of these bills and Service correspondence relating to them are in Files 4689 and 5017, PHS General Subject Files, 1897–1923, PHS Records, RG 90, NA.

38. Draft of letter from John S. Billings to Irving Fisher, April 8, 1909, in John S. Billings Papers, New York Public Library, New York, quoted in Waserman, "Quest for a National Health Department," p. 365.

39. *Health Activities Hearings, 1910–1911*, pp. 24–160.

40. Ibid., p. 66.

41. Ibid., p. 73.

42. Ibid., pp. 200–202. A membership list of prominent members is included in the record of the hearing.

43. Ibid., pp. 102–7.

44. Ibid., pp. 206–7. Morris Fishbein, in *A History of the American Medical Association, 1847–1947* (Philadelphia: W. B. Saunders Co., 1947), also stated that the league was supported by "proprietary medical interests" which had been "seriously damaged by the exposés" published in the *Journal of the American Medical Association*. See pp. 260–61.

45. *Health Activities Hearings, 1910–1911*, p. 226.

46. Ibid., p. 563.

47. Ibid., pp. 292–314.

48. Ibid., pp. 336–51; quotations are from pp. 346, 348.

49. Ibid., pp. 94, 99.

50. Ibid., pp. 94, 199–200.

51. *An Act to Change the Name of the Public Health and Marine Hospital Service, to Increase the Pay of Officers of Said Service, and for Other Purposes,* August 14, 1912, 37 *Stat. L.* 309.

52. For biographical information on Phelps see J. McKeen Cattell and Jacques Cattell, eds., *American Men of Science,* 5th ed. (New York: Science Press, 1933), p. 879. The first director of the Division of Chemistry, J. H. Kastle, resigned in 1901 and was followed by E. C. Franklin, who served from 1911 to 1913. Phelps served as director from 1913 to 1919. Franklin, who spent most of his noteworthy career at Stanford University, apparently accomplished little research at the Hygienic Laboratory. He published nothing in the Hygienic Laboratory *Bulletin* and is not mentioned in histories of the Public Health Service. After leaving the Laboratory, however, he achieved national recognition in the field of ammonia chemistry and served a term as president of the American Chemical Society. For biographical information on Franklin see Henry M. Leicester, "Edward Curtis Franklin," in Miles, ed., *American Chemists and Chemical Engineers,* pp. 158–59.

53. Williams, *USPHS,* p. 315.

54. Earle B. Phelps et al.,"A Study of the Pollution and Natural Purification of the Ohio River," *Public Health Bulletin,* no. 143 (July 1924), entire issue.

55. PHS *Annual Report,* 1913, p. 29; 1914, pp. 91, 317; 1915, p. 357; 1916, p. 369; 1917, p. 335; 1918, p. 323; 1919, p. 305; 1920, p. 363; 1921, p. 409.

56. PHS *Annual Report,* 1915, p. 17.

57. Wilson G. Smillie, *Public Health: Its Promise for the Future* (New York: Macmillan Co., 1955), p. 468.

58. The correspondence from 1913 to 1917 on these proposals and copies of the bills are in file 4689, PHS General Subject Files, 1897–1923, PHS Records, RG 90, NA.

59. For biographical information on Blue, see *American Men of Science,* 7th ed., 1944, p. 165; "Rupert Blue," *AJPH* 38: 909 (June 1948); "Rupert Blue," *JAMA* 137: 481 (May 29, 1948); Fishbein, *A History of the American Medical Association,* pp. 735–37; Williams, *USPHS,* pp. 479–81; Victoria A. Harden, "Rupert Lee Blue," in Warren F. Kuehl, ed., *Biographical Dictionary of Internationalists* (Westport, Conn.: Greenwood Press, 1983), pp. 83–85.

60. Blue's work on plague is in "The Rat and Its Relation to Public Health," *Public Health Bulletin,* no. 30 (1910), entire issue; *Reprints from the Public Health Reports,* no. 32 (May 21, 1909), no. 90 (August 16, 1912), entire issues.

61. Quoted in Furman, *Profile,* p. 283.

62. Rupert Blue, "Some of the Larger Problems of the Medical Profession," *JAMA* 66: 1899–1902 (June 17, 1916).

63. Furman, *Profile,* pp. 314–16.

64. Williams, *USPHS,* pp. 563–78.

65. *Urgent Deficiency Appropriation Act,* March 28, 1918, ch. 28, 40 *Stat.*

L. 468. These funds were augmented by subsequent appropriations: *Act of July 1, 1918*, ch. 113, 40 *Stat. L.* 645; *Act of November 4, 1918*, ch. 201, 40 *Stat. L.* 1025.

66. Williams, *USPHS*, p. 562.

67. U.S. Congress, *Joint Resolution to Establish a Reserve of the Public Health Service*, October 27, 1918, ch. 196, 40 *Stat. L.* 1017.

68. U.S. Congress, *Joint Resolution to Aid in Combatting "Spanish Influenza" and Other Communicable Diseases*, October 1, 1918, ch. 179, 40 *Stat. L.* 1008.

69. For a discussion of the pandemic see Alfred W. Crosby, Jr., *Epidemic and Peace, 1918* (Westport, Conn.: Greenwood Press, 1976).

70. Williams, *USPHS*, pp. 597–601; Furman, *Profile*, pp. 325–27.

71. PHS *Annual Report*, 1918, p. 13.

72. Ibid., pp. 60–68; Williams, *USPHS*, pp. 592–95; Furman, *Profile*, pp. 323–24.

73. U.S. President, Executive Order, July 1, 1918, cited in *United States Public Health Service Regulations, 1931* (Washington, D.C.: Government Printing Office, 1931), p. 214.

74. *Interdepartmental Social Hygiene Board*, July 9, 1918, ch. 143, 40 *Stat. L.* 886.

75. Grants had been made through the Department of Agriculture to scientists working at the Agricultural Experiment Stations. While some of this work had important medical implications—E. V. McCollum's work on nutrition, for example—it was funded for its possible contribution to agriculture, not medicine. See Charles E. Rosenberg, *No Other Gods: On Science and American Social Thought* (Baltimore: Johns Hopkins University Press, 1976), chs. 8–11.

76. PHS *Annual Report*, 1919, pp. 17–21.

77. Furman, *Profile*, p. 332.

78. An expanded discussion of this is in ch. 3.

79. Memorandum, John R. Heller, former director of the National Cancer Institute, to Wyndham Miles, February 6, 1974, copy in possession of the author.

80. PHS *Annual Report*, 1920, p. 15.

Chapter Three: Alliance with the National Health Movement

1. C.-E.A. Winslow to Thomas Parran, May 12, 1933, File "Federal Government Reorganization—Recommendations of 1933—General Correspondence," Thomas Parran Papers, University Archives, University of Pittsburgh, Pittsburgh, Pa. Hereafter cited as Parran Papers.

2. On the development of opposition by the American Medical Association to national health insurance see Ronald L. Numbers, *Almost Persuaded: American Physicians and Compulsory Health Insurance, 1912–1920* (Baltimore: Johns Hopkins University Press, 1978); James G. Burrow, *Organized Medicine in the Progressive Era: The Move toward Monopoly* (Baltimore: Johns Hopkins University Press, 1977).

3. Barbara Gutmann Rosenkrantz, "Cart before Horse: Theory, Practice and Professional Image in American Public Health, 1870–1920," *JHMAS* 29: 55–73 (January 1974).

4. For biographical information on Lord see William F. Willoughby's sketch of him in Dumas Malone, ed., *Dictionary of American Biography*, vol. 11 (New York: Charles Scribner's Sons, 1933), pp. 407–8.

5. See, for example, the memorandum from Surgeon General Hugh Cumming to Undersecretary of the Treasury Ogden Mills, dated December 27, 1929, in which Cumming explained that the "underlying objection by the Bureau of the Budget" to the Service reorganization bill was "the so-called 'militarization' of the Service," File 1220 General, PHS General Subject Files, 1924–35, PHS Records, RG 90, NA.

6. It is uncertain if Lord opposed the Public Health Service because of his religious beliefs, but Service leaders perceived that his affiliation was not helpful to them. Surgeon General Cumming wrote to William H. Welch on September 3, 1929, that "at the insistence of the then Christian Scientist Director of the Budget, President Coolidge vetoed the [Service reorganization] bill," File 1220 General, PHS General Subject Files, 1924–35, PHS Records, RG 90, NA.

7. Williams, *USPHS*, pp. 602–11.

8. Various forms of this bill were entitled *To Reorganize and Promote Efficiency of the United States Public Health Service* and were introduced as H.R. 8566, 67th Cong., 1st sess., October 10, 1921; S. 2764, 67th Cong., 1st sess., November 22, 1921; and S. 3150, 67th Cong., 2nd sess., February 14, 1922. Another bill, *To Promote the Efficiency of the United States Public Health Service*, was introduced as S. 3027, 68th Cong., 1st sess., April 7, 1924.

9. Three bills entitled *Providing for a Commissioned Status to Sanitary Engineers* were introduced as H.R. 7541, 67th Cong., 1st sess., July 1, 1921; S. 4252, 67th Cong., 4th sess., December 30, 1922; and S. 1687, 68th Cong., 1st sess., January 3, 1924.

10. M. Allen Pond, "Presidential Initiatives in Organizing Health Affairs: From Harding to Roosevelt," *Presidential Studies Quarterly* 13: 418 (Summer 1983).

11. The Veterans' Bureau became a part of the Veterans Administration when it was created in 1930.

12. Williams, *USPHS*, pp. 608–09.

13. U.S. Congress, S. Joint Resolution 191, 66th Cong., 2nd sess., December 14, 1920 quoted in James A. Tobey, "State Health Notes—Legislation," *AJPH* 11: 175 (February 1921).

14. James A. Tobey, "National Congressional Procedures," *AJPH* 11: 470 (May 1921).

15. One earlier proposal favored by the Service was the so-called Fess-Kenyon bill, introduced in 1921 (S. 1607, H.R. 5837, 67th Cong., 1st sess.). See James A. Tobey, "State Health Notes—Legislation," *AJPH* 11: 676, 681 (July 1921).

16. James A. Tobey, "State Health Notes—Legislation," *AJPH* 11: 383 (April 1921).

17. Ibid. For biographical information of Smoot see the sketch of him by Milton R. Merrill in Edward T. James, ed., *Dictionary of American Biography*, supplement 3 (New York: Charles Scribner's Sons, 1973), pp. 726–28; for biographical information on King see U.S. Congress, House, *Biographical Directory of the American Congress, 1774–1949*, House Document No. 607, 81st Cong., 2nd sess. (Washington, D.C.: Government Printing Office, 1950), p. 1237.

18. For biographical information on Cumming, see "Hugh S. Cumming," *AJPH* 39: 225 (February 1949); "Hugh S. Cumming," *JAMA* 139: 46 (January 1, 1949); Williams, *USPHS*, pp. 482–84; Victoria A. Harden, "Hugh Smith Cumming," in Kuehl, ed., *Biographical Dictionary of Internationalists*, pp. 186–87; unpublished autobiography, Hugh S. Cumming Papers, Accession Number (AN) 6922-K, Manuscripts Department, University of Virginia Library, Charlottesville; hereafter cited as Cumming Papers. Quotations from these papers are used by permission of the University of Virginia Library and of Ambassador Hugh S. Cumming, Jr.

19. Cumming's studies of the pollution of tidal waters in Maryland, Virginia, New Jersey, New York, and Delaware are in *BHL* 104 (1916), entire issue; *Reprints from the Public Health Reports* no. 181 (1914), entire issue.

20. Furman, *Profile*, pp. 329–31.

21. "Hugh Cumming," Profile section, *New York Times Magazine*, June 10, 1928, p. 17.

22. Ibid.

23. Pond, "Presidential Initiatives," p. 419.

24. "Federal Health Reorganization," *AJPH* 15: 143 (February 1925).

25. Hugh H. Young to Hugh S. Cumming, January 24, 1925, Cumming Papers, AN 6922, Box 14, folder 3.

26. Cumming to Hugh H. Young, January 17, 1925, Cumming Papers, AN 6922, Box 14, folder 3. See also Pond's discussion of this in "Presidential Initiatives," p. 420.

27. Harden, "Toward a National Institute of Health," p. 143.

28. Ibid., Figure 9, p. 145.

29. Ibid., p. 143. These figures were obtained from the personnel section of the annual reports for the years 1907–36.

30. PHS *Annual Report*, 1921, p. 13.

31. Ibid.

32. Ibid., 1922, p. 14.

33. Ibid., 1923, p. 6.

34. Ibid., 1922, p. 66.

35. For biographical information on Clark see A. Baird Hastings, "William Mansfield Clark, 1884–1964," *Year Book of the American Philosophical Society* (Philadelphia: American Philosophical Society, 1965), pp. 116–20; *Notable Contributions*, pp. 13–16; George M. Atkins, Jr., "William Mansfield Clark," in Miles, ed., *American Chemists and Chemical Engineers*, pp. 79–80.

36. William Mansfield Clark, *The Determination of Hydrogen Ions: An Elementary Treatise on the Hydrogen Electrode, Indicators, and Supplementary Methods, with an Indexed Bibliography on Applications* (Baltimore: Williams & Wilkins Co., 1920).

37. Hastings, "William Mansfield Clark," p. 118; these papers were published as "Studies on Oxidation-Reduction," *BHL* 151 (1928), entire issue.

38. National Health Council, *Statement, 1921–1925* (New York: National Health Council, 1925), p. 9.

39. Ibid., p. 4.

40. See list of officers and staff members of the National Health Council in ibid.

41. Louis I. Dublin, *A Family of Thirty Million: The Story of the Metropolitan Life Insurance Company* (New York: Metropolitan Life Insurance Co., 1943), p. 430.

42. This was one year before Eugene H. Porter, health commissioner of New York State, addressed the Association of Life Insurance Presidents at their annual meeting in Chicago and urged them to take up the cause of preventive medicine. See Porter, *The Fight Against Preventable Diseases* (Albany, N.Y.: State Department of Health, Division of Publicity and Education, n.d.), cited in George Rosen, *Preventive Medicine in the United States, 1900–1975: Trends and Interpretations* (New York: Prodist, 1977), pp. 17–18, footnote 61.

43. Dublin, *A Family of Thirty Million*, pp. 423–24

44. Rosen, *Preventive Medicine in the United States*, p. 58.

45. William Bristol Shaw, "Haley Fiske," in Allen Johnson and Dumas Malone, eds., *Dictionary of American Biography* vol. 6 (New York: Charles Scribner's Sons, 1931), pp. 419–20; U.S. Congress, House Committee on Interstate and Foreign Commerce, *Hearing before a Subcommittee of the Committee on Interstate and Foreign Commerce on H.R. 10125, to Provide for the Coordination of the Public Health Activities of the Government and for Other Purposes*, 69th Cong., 1st sess., February 24 and 25, 1927, pp. 16–17. Hereafter cited as 1927 Parker bill *Hearings*.

46. National Health Council, *Statement, 1921–1925*, pp. 9–13.

47. Information on Tobey was obtained from Dr. Tobey through correspondence and a tape-recorded interview, May 4, 1973, by Wyndham Miles and is quoted in Miles's "Further Development of the Public Health Service by the Parker Act, 1930," unpublished manuscript, National Library of Medicine, n.d., p. 2.

48. Ibid.

49. James A. Tobey, "State Health Notes—Legislation," *AJPH* 11: 470 (May 1921).

50. James A. Tobey, "Public Health Legislation," *AJPH* 14: 732 (July 1924).

51. "Progress on Federal Health Correlation," *AJPH* 20: 639 (June 1930).

52. Resolution on Federal Health Correlation adopted by the American Public Health Association at its 54th Annual Meeting, St. Louis, Mo., October 19–22, 1925, published in *AJPH* 15: 1102 (December 1925).

53. Ibid.

54. "Federal Health Reorganization," *AJPH* 15: 143–44 (February 1925).

55. James A. Tobey, *The National Government and Public Health* (Baltimore: Johns Hopkins Press, 1926), p. 384.

56. Ibid.

57. Ibid., p. 356.

58. Ibid., p. 353.

59. Ibid., p. 384.

60. Ibid., p. 385.

61. Ibid.

62. Ibid., p. 399.

63. Leigh, *Federal Health Administration*, p. 503.

64. James A. Tobey, "The Sixty-Eighth Congress," *AJPH*: 15: 383–84 (March 1925).

65. Haley Fiske to Calvin Coolidge, July 30, 1925, Cumming Papers, AN 6922, Box 14, folder 3.

66. Miles, "Further Development of the Public Health Service by the Parker Act, 1930," p. 5.

67. Hugh S. Cumming autobiography, pp. 309–10, AN 6922-K, Cumming Papers.

68. Ibid.

69. Cumming to Olin West, November 16, 1925, Cumming Papers, AN 6922, Box 14, folder 3. W. F. Willoughby was the director of the Institute for Government Research in 1925.

70. Cumming to C.-E.A. Winslow, November 18, 1925, Cumming Papers, AN 6922, Box 14, folder 3.

71. Cumming to Olin West, November 16, 1925, Cumming Papers, AN 6922, Box 14, folder 3.

72. Cumming received letters soliciting his views from the leaders of several health organizations who were preparing to discuss the proposals within their associations. See, for example, Cumming to C.-E.A. Winslow, November 18, 1925, Cumming Papers, AN 6922, Box 14, folder 3; and Cumming autobiography, p. 302, Cumming Papers, AN 6922-K.

73. Telegram, W. C. Rucker to W. C. Billings, June 1, 1925; letter from Cumming to "Dear Doctor," September 21, 1925; both in File 1220 General, Box 106, folder 3, PHS General Subject Files, 1924–35, RG 90, NA.

74. Hugh S. Cumming autobiography, p. 302, Cumming Papers, AN 6922-K.

75. James A. Tobey, *The National Government and Public Health*, pp. 395–401.

76. *AJPH* 16: 166 (February 1926).

77. Miles, "Further Development of the Public Health Service by the Parker Act, 1930," p. 13.

78. U.S. Congress, House, *A Bill to Provide for the Coordination of the Public Health Activities of the Government, and for Other Purposes,* H.R. 10125, 69th Cong., 1st sess., March 8, 1926. A copy of the bill is in *Records Regarding Coordination of Federal Public Health Activities, 1926–1929,* four notebooks; notebook one, "1925–1926," Records of the Public Health Service,

Record Group 90, National Archives, Washington, D.C. Hereafter cited as Coordination Notebooks, PHS Records, RG 90, NA.

79. Memorandum Relative to Coordination of Federal Health Activities, January 4, 1928, p. 8, File .0021, "National Institute of Health," Box 90, Records of the National Institute of Health, Records of the Public Health Service, Record Group 90, National Archives, Washington D.C. Heareafter cited as Parker Bill Explanatory Memorandum, 1928, File .0021, Box 90, NIH Records, PHS Records, RG 90, NA. A copy of this memorandum is also in notebook three, "1928," Coordination Notebooks, PHS Records, RG 90, NA. An earlier memorandum, in notebook one, "1925–1926," similarly explains the provisions of the Parker bill, but in less detail.

80. Parker Bill Explanatory Memorandum, 1928, p. 8, File .0021, Box 90, NIH Records, PHS Records, RG 90, NA.

81. Ibid., p. 5.

82. Ibid.

83. William H. Welch, in 1927 Parker Bill *Hearings*, p. 34.

84. Parker Bill Explanatory Memorandum, 1928, p. 15, Box 90, NIH Records, PHS Records, RG 90, NA.

85. Memorandum for the Secretary of the Treasury (costs), April 10, 1926; Memorandum for the Secretary of the Treasury (personnel), April 13, 1926; File 1220 General, PHS General Subject Files, 1924–35, RG 90, NA. The Coordination Notebooks also contain many sheets of estimates of the increase or decrease in cost for each employee under the Parker bill's provisions. See notebooks one, two, and three, Coordination Notebooks, PHS Records, RG 90, NA.

86. John W. Kerr initialled a memorandum on Tobey's visit, "Memorandum Relative to H.R. 10125," May 13, 1926, notebook one, "1925–1926," Coordination Notebooks, PHS Records, RG 90, NA.

87. Memorandum dated December 8, 1926, notebook one, "1925–1926," Coordination Notebooks, PHS Records, RG 90, NA.

88. James A. Tobey, "Law and Legislation," *AJPH* 16: 866 (September 1926).

89. Cumming to W. C. Rucker, August 2, 1926, Cumming Papers, AN 6922, Box 15, folder 2.

90. Memorandum, December 17, 1926, notebook one, "1925–1926," Coordination Notebooks, PHS Records, RG 90, NA.

Four: Dr. Herty Proposes an Institute for Drug Research

1. For an expanded discussion of this see George Daniels, *Science in American Society: A Social History* (New York: Alfred A. Knopf, 1971), pp. 265–81; quotations are from p. 274.

2. Dupree, *Science in the Federal Government*, p. 64.

3. Ibid., p. 55.

4. Richard H. Shryock, *American Medical Research Past and Present* (New York: Commonwealth Fund, 1947), p. 88–90.

5. On the history of the Rockefeller Institute see George W. Corner, *A*

History of the Rockefeller Institute: Origins and Growth (New York: Rockefeller Press, 1964), especially pp. 18–30; on the expansion of scientific research in medicine see Steven J. Peitzman, "Scientific Medicine in America: Some Events of Its Nativity," *Forum on Medicine* 3: 548–51, 575 (August 1979).

6. Corner, *History of the Rockefeller Institute*, pp. 30–31.

7. Glenn W. Herrick, "Some Obligations and Opportunities of Scientists in the Upbuilding of the Peace," *Science* 52: 93 (July 30, 1920).

8. Lance E. Davis and Daniel J. Kevles, "The National Research Fund: A Case Study in the Industrial Support of Academic Science," *Minerva* 12: 207–8 (April 1974).

9. On Hale and the establishment of the National Research Council see Daniel J. Kevles, "George Ellery Hale, the First World War, and the Advancement of Science in America," *Isis* 59: 427–37 (Winter 1968).

10. George Ellery Hale, "Introduction," in Robert M. Yerkes, ed., *The New World of Science: Its Development during the War* (New York: Century Co., 1920; reprint ed., Freeport, N.Y.: Books for Libraries Press, 1969), p. vii.

11. Clarence J. West, "The Chemical Warfare Service," in ibid., p. 149.

12. Ibid., p. 150.

13. "Contributions from the Chemical Warfare Service," *Journal of Industrial and Engineering Chemistry* 11: 5–12, 13–19, 93–110, 185–200, 281–96, 420–43, 513–40, 621–29, 721–23, 817–36, 1013–19, 1105–16 (1919); 12: 213–23, 1054–69 (1920). Hereafter cited as *JIEC*.

14. Daniel P. Jones, "Chemical Warfare Research during World War I: A Model of Cooperative Research," in John Parascandola and James C. Whorton, eds., *Chemistry and Modern Society: Historical Essays in Honor of Aaron J. Ihde* (Washington, D.C.: American Chemical Society, 1983), pp. 165–85.

15. Ibid., pp. 175–76.

16. Burton E. Livingston, "Constructive Scientific Research by Cooperation," *Science* 51: 277, 283 (March 19, 1920).

17. George Ellery Hale, "The Possibilities of Cooperation in Research," in Yerkes, ed., *The New World of Science*, pp. 393–94; "Cooperation in Research," *Science* 51: 149–55 (February 13, 1920); and Davis and Kevles, "The National Research Fund," pp. 208–13.

18. Arthur S. Loevenhart, "The Combat Against Syphilis," in Stieglitz, ed., *Chemistry in Medicine*, p. 672; see also Carl Voegtlin's article in this book, "A Hope of Mankind—Chemotherapy," pp. 701–20. For a discussion of Ehrlich's ideas see John Parascandola, "The Theoretical Basis of Paul Ehrlich's Chemotherapy," *JHMAS* 36: 20 (January 1981).

19. Charles Holmes Herty to J. R. Bailey, January 23, 1922, Charles Holmes Herty Papers, Box 74, folder 1, Special Collections Department, Robert W. Woodruff Library, Emory University, Atlanta, Georgia. Hereafter cited as Herty Papers.

20. Both quotations are from Charles Holmes Herty's unsigned editorial, "War Chemistry in the Alleviation of Suffering," *JIEC* 10: 673–74 (September 1918).

21. Herty to John J. Abel, August 9, 1918, Herty Papers, Box 102, folder 1.

22. John J. Abel to Charles Holmes Herty, August 17, 1918, Herty Papers, Box 102, folder 1.

23. "War Chemistry in the Alleviation of Suffering," p. 673.

24. For biographical information on Herty see Frank Cameron, "Charles Holmes Herty, 1867–1938," *Journal of the American Chemical Society* 61: 1619–24 (1939); "A Crusader," *JIEC* 30: 963–64 (September 1938); Florence Wall, "Charles H. Herty: Apostle to the South," *Chemist*, February 1932, pp. 123–31; D.H. Killeffer, "Charles Holmes Herty," in Livingston Schuyler, ed., *Dictionary of American Biography*, supplement 2 (New York: Charles Scribner's Sons, 1958), pp. 300–302; A.V.H. Morey, "Charles Holmes Herty," *JIEC* 24: 1141–42 (December 1932); David H. Wilcox, Jr., "Charles Holmes Herty," in Miles, ed., *American Chemists and Chemical Engineers*, pp. 217–18.

25. Morey, "Charles Holmes Herty," p. 1442.

26. "A Crusader," p. 963.

27. On Herty's activities as a chemical "booster" see Jeffrey Louis Sturchio, "Chemists and Industry in Modern America: Studies in the Historical Application of Science Indicators" (Ph.D. dissertation, University of Pennsylvania, 1981, pp. 39–43); examples of the genre of chemical boosterism include Edwin E. Slosson, *Creative Chemistry: Descriptive of Recent Achievements in the Chemical Industries* (New York: Century, 1919); A. S. Cushman, *Chemistry and Civilization* (Boston: R. G. Badger, 1920); Harrison E. Howe, *Chemistry in the World's Work* (New York: D. Van Nostrand, 1926); and William J. Hale, *Chemistry Triumphant: The Rise and Reign of Chemistry in a Chemical World* (Baltimore: Williams & Wilkins Co., 1932).

28. H.A.B. Dunning to Charles Holmes Herty, September 21, 1918, Herty Papers, Box 102, folder 1; interview, author with Sanford M. Rosenthal, April 13, 1981, National Institutes of Health, Bethesda, Md.

29. A. S. Loevenhart, address before the New York section of the American Chemical Society, November 8, 1918, printed in "An Institute for Cooperative Research as an Aid to the American Drug Industry," *JIEC* 10: 972 (December 1918).

30. "A Central Laboratory of Research," clipping from the *Philadelphia Public Ledger*, October 6, 1918, Herty Papers, Box 102, folder 1.

31. Herty to John J. Abel, October 23, 1918, Herty Papers, Box 102, folder 1.

32. All of the letters and addresses of the invited speakers are in "An Institute for Cooperative Research as an Aid to the American Drug Industry," *JIEC* 10: 969–76 (December 1918). For Abel's letter, see pp. 969–70.

33. Ibid., p. 973.

34. Ibid., p. 974.

35. Ibid., p. 975.

36. Ibid., p. 971.

37. Ibid., p. 973.

38. John J. Abel to Charles Holmes Herty, November 21, 1918, Herty Papers, Box 102, folder 1.

39. Minutes of the New York Section of the American Chemical Society, November 8, 1918, Herty Papers, Box 102, folder 2.

40. Ibid.

41. A minor stumbling block arose when Herty discovered that Abel was not currently a member of the American Chemical Society, a requirement for committee membership. In short order Abel's dues were submitted to remedy the problem. See correspondence in Herty Papers, Box 102, folder 2.

42. Stieglitz was not a member of the original committee but was added in April 1920. See summary "History of the Committee's Work," p. 2, prepared by Charles Holmes Herty in 1921, Herty Papers, Box 102, folder 6. John Parascandola observed that Stieglitz's appointment may have come in response to charges that an eastern establishment was monopolizing the work of the committee. See "Charles Holmes Herty and the Effort to Establish an Institute for Drug Research in Post World War I America," in Parascandola and Whorton, eds., *Chemistry and Modern Society*, pp. 90–94.

43. Edward Kremers to F. R. Eldred, December 11, 1918, Herty Papers, Box 102, folder 1.

44. Frank R. Eldred to Charles Holmes Herty, December 31, 1918, Herty Papers, Box 102, folder 1.

45. Cited in John M. Francis to Charles Holmes Herty, April 23, 1919, Herty Papers, Box 102, folder 3.

46. Ibid.

47. See John Duffy's discussion of this in *The Healers: A History of American Medicine* (Urbana: University of Illinois Press, 1976), pp. 313–14, quotation from p. 314; James G. Burrow, *AMA: Voice of American Medicine* (Baltimore: Johns Hopkins Press, 1963), pp. 27–53; Fishbein, *A History of the American Medical Association*, pp. 197–213, 1018–20.

48. On the establishment of the Council on Pharmacy and Chemistry, see Burrow, *AMA: Voice of American Medicine*, pp. 107–31; and Fishbein, *A History of the American Medical Association*, pp. 235–36.

49. Parascandola, "Charles Holmes Herty and the Effort to Establish an Institute for Drug Research," pp. 90–94.

50. Herty to J. M. Francis, May 2, 1919, Herty Papers, Box 102, folder 3. The offending article was, according to Herty, written by Dr. Paul Nicholas Leech of the AMA's laboratory.

51. Eldred to Charles Holmes Herty, March 5, 1919, Herty Papers, Box 102, folder 3.

52. Ibid.

53. Ibid.

54. Herty to Frank R. Eldred, March 12, 1919, Herty Papers, Box 102, folder 3.

55. Herty to John J. Abel, February 25, 1919, Herty Papers, Box 102, folder 2.

56. Ibid.

57. Committee report, March 15, 1919, Herty Papers, Box 102, folder 3.

58. Jacques Loeb, *The Mechanistic Conception of Life* (Chicago: University of Chicago Press, 1912).

59. Committee report, March 15, 1919, Herty Papers, Box 102, folder 3.

60. J. M. Francis to Charles Holmes Herty, April 23, 1919, Herty Papers, Box 102, folder 3.

61. Edward Marshall, interview with Charles Holmes Herty, released February 23, 1919, p. 5; Herty Papers, Box 102, folder 2.

62. The American Drug Manufacturers Association endorsement is noted in the summary "History of the Committee's Work," p. 2, prepared by Charles Holmes Herty in 1921, Herty Papers, Box 102, folder 6; see letter from Henry A. Christian of the Medical Sciences Division to Herty on the National Research Council's resolution, February 2, 1920, Herty Papers, Box 102, folder 4.

63. For biographical information on Garvan see Arthur W. Hixson, "Francis P. Garvan, 1875–1937," *JIEC*, News Edition 15: 539–40 (December 20, 1937); Charles Holmes Herty, "Advance of the Nation through the Science of Chemistry," *Journal of Chemical Education* 6: 1037–44 (June 1929); obituary, *New York Times*, November 8, 1937, p. 23.

64. Hixson, "Francis P. Garvan," p. 539.

65. Herty, "Advance of the Nation through the Science of Chemistry," p. 1037.

66. For information on the Chemical Foundation see [Edward Muh], "The Chemical Foundation, Inc.," 2 vols., typescript, ca. 1954, in the Francis P. Garvan Estate Collection, Small File No. 13 (American Heritage Center, Coe Library, University of Wyoming, Laramie); "Prospectus" of the Chemical Foundation, Herty Papers, Box 108, folder 6; Williams Haynes, *American Chemical Industry*, 6 vols. (New York: D. Van Nostrand, 1945–54), 3: 270–71; and *Aims and Purposes of the Chemical Foundation, Incorporated, and the Reasons for Its Organization* (New York: Chemical Foundation, 1919).

67. "Prospectus" of the Chemical Foundation, Herty Papers, Box 108, folder 6.

68. The monograph series was inaugurated with the report of Charles Holmes Herty's committee (discussed later in the text), *The Future Independence and Progress of American Medicine in the Age of Chemistry* (New York: Chemical Foundation, 1921); others in the series included Harrison E. Howe, ed., *Chemistry in Industry: A Cooperative Work Intended to Give Examples of the Contributions Made to Industry by Chemistry*, 2 vols. (New York: Chemical Foundation, 1924–25); Joseph S. Chamberlain and C. A. Brown, eds., *Chemistry in Agriculture: A Cooperative Work Intended to Give Examples of the Contributions Made to Agriculture by Chemistry* (New York: Chemical Foundation, 1926); and Stieglitz, ed., *Chemistry in Medicine*.

69. Hixson, "Francis P. Garvan," p. 539. Because of his generous personal support for chemistry in a variety of ways, Garvan was awarded in 1929 the American Chemical Society's Priestly Medal. The third recipient of the triennial medal, Garvan remains the only layperson ever to receive the award.

70. Herty to committee members, September 30, 1920, Herty Papers, Box 102, folder 4.

71. Minutes of the Joint Meeting of the Committee on an Institute for Drug Research and Representatives of the Chemical Foundation, Inc., October 11, 1920, Herty Papers, Box 102, folder 4.

72. Herty to American Chemical Society President Edgar F. Smith, January 26, 1921, Herty Papers, Box 102, folder 5.

73. Ibid.; Edgar F. Smith to Charles Holmes Herty, January 27, 1921, Herty Papers, Box 102, folder 5.

74. H. Gideon Wells to Charles Holmes Herty, December 8, 1919, Herty Papers, Box 102, folder 3.

75. Treat B. Johnson to Charles Holmes Herty, November 29, 1920, Box 102, folder 4.

76. See, for example the letters from William J. Mayo of the Mayo Clinic and George E. Vincent of the Rockefeller Foundation, printed in later hearings on the bill in U.S. Congress, Senate Committee on Commerce, *Proposed National Institute of Health*, Senate Rept. 1280, 70th Cong., 1st sess., May 3 (calendar day, May 25), 1928, pp. 76–78. Hereafter cited as 1928 Ransdell bill *Hearings*. All page citations are taken from the copy of the hearings included in this Senate report.

77. Johnson to Julius Stieglitz, March 7, 1921, Herty Papers, Box 102, folder 5.

78. Herty et al., *The Future Independence and Progress of American Medicine in the Age of Chemistry*, p. 80.

79. Herty to committee members January 27, 1922, Herty Papers, Box 102, folder 7.

80. Ibid.

81. Draft report of the Chemical Foundation's work, Herty Papers, Box 102, folder 8.

82. Herty to committee members, January 27, 1922, Herty Papers, Box 102, folder 7.

83. Herty et al., *The Future Independence and Progress of American Medicine in the Age of Chemistry*, p. 66.

84. "The Future Independence and Progress of American Medicine in the Age of Chemistry," *JAMA* 78: 807 (March 18, 1922); see also Julius Stieglitz's comment on the review in his letter to Charles Holmes Herty, March 11, 1922, Herty Papers, Box 102, folder 7.

85. Copy of petition attached to letter from Frank O. Taylor to Charles Holmes Herty, April 19, 1922, Herty Papers, Box 102, folder 7.

86. Harvey L. Curtis to Charles Holmes Herty, October 25, 1922, Herty Papers, Box 102, folder 7.

87. Taylor to Charles Holmes Herty, April 19, 1922, Herty Papers, Box 102, folder 7.

88. Memorandum, May 10, 1924, File 1220 General, PHS General Subject Files, 1924–35, PHS Records, RG 90, NA.

89. Andrew Mellon to L. Heisler Ball, May 29, 1924, File 1220 General, PHS General Subject Files, 1924–35, PHS Records, RG 90, NA.

90. Charles Holmes Herty, Postscript to Report of the Committee on an Institute for Chemo-Medical Research to the President of the American Chemical Society, April 7, 1924, Herty Papers, Box 102, folder 8.

91. Report of the Committee on an Institute for Chemo-Medical Research, March 18, 1925, Herty Papers, Box 102, folder 8.

92. See, for example, the discussion of Frederick T. Gate's efforts to raise funds for institutions such as the University of Chicago in Ettling, *Germ of Laziness*, pp. 64–72.

93. William A. Wilcox to James F. Norris, September 13, 1926; Herty to Wilcox, September 25, 1926, Herty Papers, Box 102, folder 9.

Five: Turning to Uncle Sam

1. Arthur Meier Schlesinger, *The Rise of Modern America, 1865–1951* (New York: Macmillan Co., 1951), p. 291.

2. George Brown Tindall, *America: A Narrative History* (New York: W. W. Norton & Co., 1984), p. 1028.

3. James A. Tobey, "Legislation-Federal," *AJPH* 11: 1104 (December 1921); Davis and Kevles, "National Research Fund," p. 219, note 35.

4. Charles Holmes Herty to John M. Francis, May 2, 1919, Herty Papers, Box 102, folder 3.

5. Shryock, *American Medical Research*, p. 81.

6. The years 1915 through 1935 came to be known as the "doldrum years" in chemotherapy. See Harry F. Dowling, *Fighting Infection: Conquests of the Twentieth Century* (Cambridge, Mass.: Harvard University Press, 1977), pp. 105–7.

7. For an example of the arguments of those who opposed cooperative research see R. A. Harper, "The Stimulation of Research after the War," *Science* 51: 473–78 (May 14, 1920).

8. Callie Hull, comp., "Funds Available in 1920 in the United States for the Encouragement of Scientific Research," *Bulletin of the National Research Council*, no. 9 (March 1921); Callie Hull and Clarence J. West, comps., "Funds Available in the United States for the Support and Encouragement of Research in Science and Its Technologies," 2nd ed., *Bulletin of the National Research Council*, no. 66 (November, 1928); Hull and West, comps., "Funds Available in Science and Its Technologies," 3rd ed., *Bulletin of the National Research Council*, no. 95 (June 1934). Hereafter cited as NRC *Bulletin*. The methods used in analyzing these data are in Harden, "Toward a National Institute of Health," Appendix A, pp. 343–53.

9. Hull and West, "Funds Available in the United States for the Support and Encouragement of Research in Science and Its Technologies," p. 44.

10. In 1920 only two firms made awards; in 1928 fourteen did; and in 1934 thirty did. Some firms donated funds in more than one year; thus the total number of separate firms contributing was forty-three. My counts from NRC *Bulletin* nos. 9, 66, 95.

11. For a breakdown of the amounts expended in different medical categories by year, see Harden, "Toward a National Institute of Health," Tables 3–5, Appendix A, pp. 349–53.

12. Robert E. Kohler, "Warren Weaver and the Rockefeller Foundation Program in Molecular Biology: A Case Study in the Management of Science," in Nathan Reingold, ed., *The Sciences in the American Context: New Per-*

spectives (Washington, D.C.: Smithsonian Institution Press, 1979), pp. 249–93.

13. U.S. Bureau of the Census, *Historical Statistics of the United States, Colonial Times to 1970* (Washington, D.C.: Government Printing Office, 1976), pp. 210–11.

14. "Registration in American Universities," *Science* 69: 45–47 (January 11, 1929).

15. Stanley Cohen, "American Foundations as Patrons of Science: The Commitment to Individual Research," in Reingold, ed., *The Sciences in the American Context*, pp. 229–47.

16. Ronald C. Tobey, *The American Ideology of National Science, 1919–1930* (Pittsburgh: University of Pittsburgh Press, 1971), pp. 6–7.

17. Lafayette B. Mendel, "Some Tendencies in the Promotion of Chemical Research," *Science* 65: 559 (June 10, 1927).

18. For one example, see H. P. Cody, "The Chemistry of the Future," *Science* 65: 1–4 (January 1927).

19. President's Research Committee on Social Trends, *Recent Social Trends in the United States*, 2 vols. (New York: McGraw-Hill Book Co., 1933), 1: 393.

20. Paul Starr, *The Social Transformation of American Medicine* (New York: Basic Books, 1982), pp. 3–21. Richard Shryock also discussed this trend; see his *The Development of Modern Medicine: An Interpretation of the Social and Scientific Factors Involved* (New York: Alfred A. Knopf, 1936; reprint ed., Madison: University of Wisconsin Press, 1974), pp. 336–55.

21. Robert S. Lynd and Helen M. Lynd, *Middletown: A Study in American Culture* (New York: Harcourt, Brace, & Co., 1929), pp. 189–91; quotation from p. 191.

22. Irving Fisher and Eugene Lyman Fisk, *How to Live: Rules for Healthful Living Based on Modern Science* (New York: Funk & Wagnalls Co., 1915; 18th ed., rev., 1926). For an analysis of this genre see John C. Burnham, "Change in the Popularization of Health in the United States," *BHM* 58: 183–97 (Summer 1984), especially pp. 186–88.

23. Davis and Kevles, "The National Research Fund," pp. 215–20.

24. On the establishment of the National Science Foundation see J. Merton England, *A Patron for Pure Science: The National Science Foundation's Formative Years, 1945–57* (Washington, D.C.: National Science Foundation, 1982).

25. Herty to committee members, March 22, 1926, Herty Papers, Box 102, folder 9.

26. Herty to Joseph E. Ransdell, January 19, 1926, Herty Papers, Box 103, folder 3.

27. Joseph E. Ransdell to Charles Holmes Herty, February 27, 1926, Herty Papers, Box 103, folder 3.

28. Herty to committee members, March 22, 1926, Herty Papers, Box 102, folder 9.

29. Treat B. Johnson to Charles Holmes Herty, March 24, 1926, Herty Papers, Box 102, folder 9.

30. F. O. Taylor to Charles Holmes Herty, March 26, 1926, Herty Papers, Box 102, folder 9.

31. Raymond Bacon to Charles Holmes Herty, March 24, 1926, Herty Papers, Box 102, folder 9.

32. Julius Stieglitz to Charles Holmes Herty, March 26, 1926, Herty Papers, Box 102, folder 9.

33. C. L. Alsberg to Charles Holmes Herty, March 30, 1926, Herty Papers, Box 102, folder 9.

34. For biographical information on Ransdell see Adras P. Laborde, *A National Southerner: Ransdell of Louisiana* (New York: Benziger, 1951); George Quitman Flynn, "Senator Joseph E. Ransdell of Louisiana and the Underwood Tariff of 1913" (M.A. thesis, Louisiana State University, 1962); Frederick W. Williamson and George T. Goodman, eds., *Eastern Louisiana: A History of the Watershed of the Quachita River and the Florida Parishes*, 3 vols. (Louisville: Historical Records Association, 1939), 3: 586 ff; "Joseph Eugene Ransdell," *Biographical Directory of the American Congress, 1774–1961* (Washington, D.C.: Government Printing Office, 1961), p. 1498.

35. LaBorde, *National Southerner*, p. 17.

36. Quoted in LaBorde, *National Southerner*, p. 69.

37. For an account of the establishment of the National Leprosarium see Furman, *Profile*, pp. 347–49.

38. Memorandum, Charles Holmes Herty to Francis Garvan, February 9, 1927, Herty Papers, Box 103, folder 4.

39. Ransdell to Charles Holmes Herty, April 2, 1926, Herty Papers, Box 103, folder 3.

40. Herty to Joseph E. Ransdell, April 10, 1926, Herty Papers, Box 103, folder 3.

41. Ransdell to Charles Holmes Herty, June 1, 1926, Herty Papers, Box 103, folder 3.

42. Memorandum, Ralph C. Williams to Carlton B. Chapman, July 28, 1969, copy in possession of the author. Williams was Kerr's assistant in 1926. He recalled seeing Kerr "labor for several weeks" preparing the first draft of the legislation, and commented that "much of the detail was based on the judgement of Dr. Kerr and Senator Ransdell, with suggestions from Dr. [Lewis R.] Thompson."

43. U.S. Congress, Senate, *A Bill to Establish a National Institute of Health, to Authorize Increased Appropriations for the Hygienic Laboratory, and to Authorize the Government to Accept Donations for Use in Ascertaining the Cause, Prevention, and Cure of Disease Affecting Human Beings*, S. 4540, 69th Cong., 1st sess., July 1, 1926. A copy of the bill is in the Herty Papers, Box 104, folder 8.

44. See typescript of speech in Herty Papers, Box 104, folder 8. The name was to prove more advantageous than Herty's term *chemo-medical* research institute. Herty wrote to Ransdell in 1930, "You were wise in insisting on that name." See Herty to Joseph E. Ransdell, July 25, 1930, Herty Papers, Box 104, folder 4.

45. U.S. Congress, Senate, *Congressional Record*, 69th Cong., 1st sess., July 2, 1926, pp. 12650, 12652.

46. Ibid., p. 12647.

47. See ch. 2 for a discussion of this.

48. 1928 Ransdell bill *Hearings*, p. 72.

49. Ellis W. Hawley, "Herbert Hoover, the Commerce Secretariat, and the Vision of an 'Associative State,' 1921–1928," *Journal of American History* 61: 116–40 (June 1974).

50. "Chemistry and Disease," *New York Times*, July 7, 1926, p. 24.

Six: Vision and Reality in New Era Politics

1. "The Washington Session," *JAMA* 88: 1716 (May 28, 1927).

2. Calvin Coolidge, *The Price of Freedom: Speeches and Addresses* (New York: Charles Scribner's Sons, 1924), p. 58.

3. "The President Signs the Lye Bill," *JAMA* 88: 926 (March 19, 1927).

4. *New York State Department of Health Monthly Bulletin* 9: 45 (1914).

5. Coolidge, *Price of Freedom*, pp. 44–45.

6. "Wants Government to Lead Health Work: Dr. C. H. Herty Advocates Creation of Research Department to Combat Disease," *New York Times*, September 26, 1926, II, p. 2.

7. Charles Holmes Herty to Joseph E. Ransdell, July 17, 1926, Herty Papers, Box 103, folder 4; Hugh Cumming to C. H. Lavinder, August 19, 1926, Cumming Papers, AN 6922, Box 15, folder 4. The quotation is from the Cumming letter discussing the proposed conference.

8. Cumming to C. H. Lavinder, August 19, 1926, Cumming Papers, AN 6922, Box 15, folder 4.

9. Cumming to Joseph E. Ransdell, September 27, 1926, Herty Papers, Box 103, folder 3.

10. Joseph E. Ransdell to Charles Holmes Herty, November 10, 1926, Herty Papers, Box 103, folder 3.

11. Hugh S. Cumming autobiography, p. 386, Cumming Papers, AN 6922-K.

12. Wyndham Miles, "Establishment of the National Institute of Health, 1930," unpublished manuscript, National Library of Medicine, n.d., p. 16.

13. A. M. Stimson, Comment on S. 4540, n.d., File OD, .0221, National Institute of Health, Records of the Public Health Service, Record Group 90, National Archives, Washington, D.C. Hereafter cited as File OD, .0221, NIH, PHS Records, RG 90, NA.

14. R. E. Dyer, Memorandum on S. 4540, August 28, 1926, File OD, .0221, NIH, PHS Records, RG 90, NA.

15. George W. McCoy, "Memorandum on Bills to Provide a National Institute of Health," March 16, 1929, File OD, .0221, NIH, PHS Records, RG 90, NA.

16. Andrew Mellon to Wesley Jones, January 8, 1927, File "S. 4540, 69th

Congress, National Institute of Health," Box 265, Series 21.2, Bureau of the Budget, U.S. Treasury Department Records, Record Group 51, National Archives, Washington, D.C. It was the practice of the Budget Bureau to assemble all information on one bill under its original congressional number; therefore all subsequent information on the Ransdell bill is in this file. Hereafter cited as File "S. 4540, 69th Cong., NIH," Box 265, Series 21.2, Budget Bureau, Treasury Dept. Records, RG 51, NA.

17. Memorandum, Charles H. Fullaway to H. M. Lord, January 26, 1927, File "S. 4540, 69th Cong., NIH," Box 265, Series 21.2, Budget Bureau, Treasury Dept. Records, RG 51, NA.

18. Memorandum, Charles Holmes Herty to Francis Garvan, February 9, 1927, Herty Papers, Box 103, folder 4.

19. Memorandum, Charles Holmes Herty to Francis Garvan, March 4, 1927, Herty Papers, Box 103, folder 4.

20. U.S., Congress, Senate, *A Bill to Establish a National Institute of Health, to Authorize Increased Appropriations for the Hygienic Laboratory, and to Authorize the Government to Accept Donations for Use in Ascertaining the Cause, Prevention, and Cure of Diseases Affecting Human Beings, and for Other Purposes*, S. 5835, 69th Cong., 2nd sess., March 2, 1927. A copy of the bill is in the Herty Papers, Box 104, folder 9.

21. H. M. Lord to Undersecretary of the Treasury G. B. Winston, January 8, 1927, notebook two, "1927," Coordination Notebooks, PHS Records, RG 90, NA.

22. President Coolidge's moniker, "Silent Cal" was never more appropriate than during the debates on the Ransdell and Parker bills. Proponents of both bills tried repeatedly to ascertain his views and whether the information conveyed by H. M. Lord was an accurate reflection of the President's feelings. They were not alone, however. Donald McCoy, in *Calvin Coolidge: The Quiet President* (New York: Macmillan Co., 1969), p. 194, quoted W. E. Brinkley as observing that the way Coolidge informed Congress on affairs of state was "so formal and perfunctory that sometimes it was difficult or impossible for Congress to discover his views." See Brinkley, *The Power of the President* (Garden City, N.Y., 1937), p. 244.

23. Memorandum Relative to H.R. 10125, January 14, 1927, initialled JWK [John Kerr], notebook two, "1927," Coordination Notebooks, PHS Records, RG 90, NA.

24. Kerr prepared a three-page list of potential witnesses. See notebook two, "1927," Coordination Notebooks, PHS Records, RG 90, NA.

25. Telegrams, Hugh S. Cumming to various witnesses, requesting their presence at breakfast meeting at Cosmos Club, February 23, 1927; Cumming to Haley Fiske, Cumming to Edgar Wood, Telegrams requesting a meeting just before hearings convened, February 23, 1927; all in File 1220 General, Box 107, folder 6, PHS General Subject Files, 1924–35, PHS Records, RG 90, NA.

26. 1927 Parker bill *Hearings*, p. 17.

27. Ibid., pp. 55–57.

28. Ibid., p. 56.

29. Ibid., pp. 64–65.

30. Ibid., pp. 66–67.

31. Ibid., pp. 30, 32.

32. Ibid., p. 36.

33. Ibid., p. 46.

34. Ibid.

35. Ibid., p. 48.

36. Ibid.

37. Ibid., p. 43.

38. Ibid., p. 68.

39. Ibid., p. 44.

40. Ibid., p. 46.

41. Cumming to Rupert Blue, May 26, 1927, Cumming Papers, AN 6922, Box 16, folder 1.

42. Herty to C. C. Pierce, May 3, 1927; Herty to Joseph E. Ransdell, May 3, 1927, Herty Papers Box 103, folder 5.

43. C. C. Pierce to Charles Holmes Herty, May 5, 1927, Herty Papers, Box 103, folder 5.

44. Herty to C. C. Pierce, May 11, 1927, Herty Papers, Box 103, folder 5.

45. Telegram, Charles Holmes Herty to Joseph E. Ransdell, May 24, 1927, Herty Papers, Box 103, folder 5.

46. Memorandum, Charles Holmes Herty to Francis Garvan, October 17, 1927, Herty Papers, Box 103, folder 5.

47. See Hugh S. Cumming's remarks on Kerr's illness in a letter to Rupert Blue, May 26, 1927, Cumming Papers, AN 6922, Box 16, folder 1.

48. Memorandum re: H.R. 10125, "Contacts with Congressmen," initialled TP [Thomas Parran], October 22, 1927, notebook two, "1927," Coordination Notebooks, PHS Records, RG 90, NA.

49. Ibid.

50. Herty to Joseph E. Ransdell, October 28, 1927, Herty Papers, Box 103, folder 5.

51. Edward Marshall to Charles Holmes Herty, November 26, 1927, Herty Papers, Box 103, folder 5.

52. Charles Holmes Herty, quoted in U.S. Congress, Senate, *Congressional Record*, 70th Cong., 1st sess., January 4, 1928, p. 946.

53. Memorandum, Charles Holmes Herty to Francis Garvan, January 10, 1928, Herty Papers, Box 103, folder 6.

54. Ibid.

55. Carl Mapes quoted in Memorandum re: H.R. 10125, initialled TP [Thomas Parran], November 21, 1927, notebook two, "1927," Coordination Notebooks, PHS Records, RG 90, NA.

56. Memorandum re: H.R. 5766, initialled TP [Thomas Parran], January 5, 1928, notebook three, "1928," Coordination Notebooks, PHS Records, RG 90, NA.

57. Memorandum re: H.R. 5766, January 7, 1928; Memorandum re: H.R. 5766, initialled TP [Thomas Parran], January 9, 1928, notebook three, "1928," Coordination Notebooks, PHS Records, RG 90, NA.

58. Memorandum re: H.R. 5766, initialled TP [Thomas Parran], January 9, 1928, notebook three, "1928," Coordination Notebooks, PHS Records, RG 90, NA.

59. U.S. Congress, House Committee on Interstate and Foreign Commerce, *Hearing before a Subcommittee of the Committee on Interstate and Foreign Commerce on H.R. 5766 to Provide for the Coordination of the Public Health Activities of the Government and for Other Purposes*, 70th Cong., 1st sess., January 11, 1928, pp. 1, 13–14, 23. Hereafter cited as 1928 Parker bill *Hearings*.

60. Ibid., p. 2.

61. Ibid., p. 6. On the certified milk movement see Manfred J. Waserman, "Henry L. Coit and the Certified Milk Movement in the Development of Modern Pediatrics," *BHM* 46: 359–90 (July–August, 1972).

62. Alice C. Evans, "Studies on *Brucella (alkaligenes melitensis),*" *BHL* 143 (August 1925); Evans, "Malta Fever: Cattle Suggested as a Possible Source of Infection, following a Serological Study of Human Serums," *Reprints from the Public Health Reports* no. 906 (March 14, 1924). Undulant fever was the human form of abortive fever in cattle; Evans correctly identified the organism that caused this disease as a variant of the same organism that caused the more virulent Malta fever in humans.

63. 1928 Parker bill *Hearings*, pp. 8–12.

64. Ibid., p. 10.

65. Ibid.

66. Ibid., pp. 39–41.

67. Ibid., pp. 31–34.

68. Telegram, C. H. Bierman to Hugh S. Cumming, February 25, 1927, Box 105, folder 4, File 1220 General, PHS General Subject Files, 1924–35, PHS Records, RG 90, NA.

69. 1928 Parker bill *Hearings*, p. 32.

70. U.S. Congress, House, *Congressional Record*, 70th Cong., 1st sess., March 7, 1928, p. 4265.

71. Ibid.

72. U.S. Congress, House, *A Bill to Provide for the Coordination of the Public Health Activities of the Government and for Other Purposes*, H.R. 10126, 70th Cong., 1st sess., February 15, 1928. A copy of H.R. 10126 and a confidential committee print of the old version of the bill, H.R. 5766, with indicated changes are in notebook three, "1928," Coordination Notebooks, PHS Records, RG 90, NA.

73. U.S. Congress, House, *Coordination of Public Health Activities of the Government*, House Rept. 733 to Accompany H.R. 10126, 70th Cong., 1st sess., February 21, 1928, p. 3.

74. Herty to Joseph E. Ransdell, January 20, 1928, Herty Papers, Box 103, folder 6.

75. Herty to Francis Garvan, February 29, 1928, Herty Papers, Box 103, folder 6.

76. Ibid.

77. Telegram, Joseph E. Ransdell to Charles Holmes Herty, Telegram, February 14, 1928, Herty Papers, Box 103, folder 6.

78. Herty to Francis Garvan, February 29, 1928, Herty Papers, Box 103, folder 3.

79. Memorandum re: Parker Bill and Ransdell Bill, initialled TP [Thomas Parran], February 18, 1928, notebook three, "1928," Coordination Notebooks, PHS Records, RG 90, NA.

80. Memorandum re: H.R. 10126 and the Ransdell Bill, initialled TP [Thomas Parran], February 23, 1928, notebook three, "1928," Coordination Notebooks, PHS Records, RG 90, NA.

81. U.S. Congress, Senate, *A Bill to Establish a National Institute of Health, to Authorize Increased Appropriations for the Hygienic Laboratory, and to Authorize the Government to Accept Donations for Use in Ascertaining the Cause, Prevention, and Cure of Diseases Affecting Human Beings, and for Other Purposes*, S. 3391, 70th Cong., 1st sess., February 27, 1928. A copy of the bill is in the Herty Papers, Box 104, folder 9.

82. Joseph E. Ransdell, quoted in Charles Holmes Herty to Francis Garvan, February 29, 1928, Herty Papers, Box 103, folder 3.

83. U.S. Congress, House, *Congressional Record*, 70th Cong., 1st sess., March 7, 1928, p. 4263.

84. Ibid., p. 4267.

85. Ibid.

86. Ibid., p. 4268.

87. Ibid., p. 4269.

88. Ibid., pp. 4271–73.

89. Cumming to Charles Holmes Herty, March 10, 1928, Herty Papers, Box 103, folder 7.

90. Ransdell to Charles Holmes Herty, April 5, 1928, Herty Papers, Box 103, folder 7.

91. Ransdell to Charles Holmes Herty, March 30, 1928, Herty Papers, Box 103, folder 7.

92. Herty to Joseph E. Ransdell, April 2, 1928, Herty Papers, Box 103, folder 7.

93. 1928 Ransdell bill *Hearings*, pp. 76–93.

94. Ibid., pp. 16–20.

95. Ibid., p. 16.

96. Ibid., p. 29.

97. Ibid., p. 35.

98. Ibid., p. 78.

99. Ibid., p. 71.

100. Ibid., p. 68.

101. Ibid., p. 23.

102. Ibid., p. 26.

103. Ibid.

104. Ibid., p. 51.

105. Ibid., p. 60.

106. Ibid., pp. 20, 21.

107. Ibid., p. 55.

108. Ibid., p. 48.

109. Ibid., p. 54.

110. Ibid., p. 53.

111. Ibid., p. 10.

112. Ibid.

113. Ransdell to Charles Holmes Herty, April 29, 1928, Herty Papers, Box 103, folder 7.

114. Ransdell to Charles Holmes Herty, May 18, 1928, Herty Papers, Box 103, folder 7.

115. U.S. Congress, Senate, S. Rept. 1280 to Accompany S. 4518, 70th Cong., 1st sess., May 25, 1928. A copy of S. 4518 is in the Herty Papers, Box 104, folder 9.

116. Herty to Mildred E. Reeves, May 29, 1928, Herty Papers, Box 103, folder 8.

117. U.S. Congress, Senate, *Congressional Record*, 70th Cong., 1st sess., May 29, 1928, p. 10601.

118. Herty to Joseph E. Ransdell, June 5, 1928, Herty Papers, Box 103, folder 8.

119. Ransdell to Charles Holmes Herty, June 6, 1928, Herty Papers, Box 103, folder 8.

120. A copy of H.R. 10126 with attached changes labeled "Original draft of Amendments agreed upon with Senator Smoot" is in notebook three, "1928," Coordination Notebooks, PHS Records, RG 90, NA.

121. U.S. Congress, Senate, *Congressional Record*, 70th Cong., 1st sess., April 24, 1928, p. 7082.

122. Ibid., May 10, 1928, p. 8340.

123. Calvin Coolidge, "Coordination of Public Health Activities in the Government," Veto Message to Accompany H.R. 10126, May 18, 1928. Quoted portions of the message are taken from S. Rept. 101 to Accompany S. 3167, 71st Cong., 2nd sess., January 18, 1930, pp. 1–2.

124. Ibid.

125. Memorandum, unsigned, May 10, 1928, notebook three, "1928," Coordination Notebooks, PHS Records, RG 90, NA. Cumming remembered this veto bitterly in later years. See his comments, Cumming autobiography, p. 314, Cumming papers, AN 6922-K.

126. James A. Tobey, "Triumph Deferred," *AJPH* 18: 949 (July 1928).

127. Ibid.

Seven: Perseverance, Compromise, and Success

1. "Association News," *AJPH* 18: 1399 (November 1928).

2. Charles Holmes Herty to Joseph E. Ransdell, May 31, 1928, Herty Papers, Box 103, folder 8.

3. Joseph E. Ransdell to Charles Holmes Herty, June 1, 1928, Herty Papers, Box 103, folder 8.

4. Herty to Florence Fabre-Rajotte, March 27, 1928, Herty Papers, Box 103, folder 7.

5. Herty to Mary F. Goldberger, April 19, 1928, Herty Papers, Box 103, folder 7.

6. Mary F. Goldberger to Charles Holmes Herty, April 16, 1928, Herty Papers, Box 103, folder 7.

7. Herty to Grace Crocker, May 29, 1928, Herty Papers, Box 103, folder 8.

8. James Harvey Young, *The Medical Messiahs: A Social History of Health Quackery in the Twentieth Century* (Princeton: Princeton University Press, 1967), p. 35; Edward L. Bernays, *Propaganda* (New York: Horace Liveright, 1928), p. 116–17; Anne Firor Scott, "On Seeing and Not Seeing: A Case of Historical Invisibility," *Journal of American History* 71: 18 (June 1984).

9. Herty to E. C. Franklin, July 21, 1928, Herty Papers, Box 103, folder 8; the plank was reprinted in U.S. Congress, Senate, *Congressional Record*, 70th Cong., 2nd sess., February 6, 1929, p. 2905.

10. Herty to E. C. Franklin, July 21, 1928, Herty Papers, Box 103, folder 8.

11. Ibid.

12. Hawley, "Herbert Hoover, the Commerce Secretariat, and the Vision of an 'Associative State,' 1921–1928," p. 134. For an excellent recent biography of Hoover see Joan Hoff Wilson, *Herbert Hoover: Forgotten Progressive*, The Library of America Biography Series (Boston: Little, Brown & Co., 1975).

13. Hawley, "Herbert Hoover, the Commerce Secretariat, and the Vision of an 'Associative State,' 1921–1928," pp. 133–134.

14. Herbert Hoover, "The Nation and Science," Address before the Society of Sigma Xi and the American Association for the Advancement of Science, Philadelphia, Pa., December 28, 1926, printed in *Science* 65: 26–28 (January 4, 1927); quotation from p. 27.

15. U.S. Presidents, *Inaugural Addresses of the American Presidents: From Washington to Kennedy*, annotated by Davis Newton Lott (New York: Holt, Rinehart, & Winston, 1961), p. 226.

16. Hugh S. Cumming to William H. Welch, September 3, 1929, File 1220 General, PHS General Subject Files, 1924–35, PHS Records, RG 90, NA. Cumming also compared conditions under Presidents Hoover and Warren G. Harding. During the Harding administration, he said, "we were constantly on the defensive about having our marbles stolen," whereas under Hoover "there seems to be an opportunity for a rather general advance." See Cumming to J. D. Long, January 28, 1930, Cumming Papers, AN 6922, Box 18, folder 3.

17. Ransdell to Charles Holmes Herty, September 12, 1928, Herty Papers, Box 103, folder 9.

18. Ransdell to Charles Holmes Herty, September 13, 1928, Herty Papers, Box 103, folder 9.

19. Ransdell to Charles Holmes Herty, September 14, 1928, Herty Papers, Box 103, folder 9.

20. Herty to Francis Garvan, October 24, 1928, Herty Papers, Box 103, folder 9.

21. Ransdell to Charles Holmes Herty, September 14, 1928, Herty Papers, Box 103, folder 9.

22. Charles H. Fullaway to H. M. Lord, November 7, 1928, File "S. 4540, 69th Cong., NIH," Box 265, Series 21.2, Budget Bureau, Treasury Department Records, RG 51, NA.

23. Ransdell to Charles Holmes Herty, November 5, 1928, Herty Papers, Box 103, folder 9.

24. Ransdell to Charles Holmes Herty, October 3, 1928, Herty Papers, Box 103, folder 9.

25. Herty to Joseph E. Ransdell, October 12, 1928, Herty Papers, Box 103, folder 9. Calvin Coolidge, Jr. died as a result of a streptococcal infection against which there was no effective treatment. A decade later, Franklin Delano Roosevelt's son would be saved dramatically from a similar infection by the newly introduced sulfanilamide.

26. Franklin Hobbs to Charles Holmes Herty, October 25 and November 23, 1928, Herty Papers, Box 103 folder 9.

27. Herty to Franklin Hobbs, December 4, 1928, Herty Papers, Box 103, folder 9.

28. Hobbs to Charles Holmes Herty, December 6, 1928, Herty Papers, Box 103, folder 9. Continued efforts to win Coolidge's support are documented in Hobbs to Calvin Coolidge, December 12, 1928, and in Telegram, Joseph E. Ransdell to Charles Holmes Herty, December 19, 1928, Herty Papers, Box 103, folder 9.

29. Telegram, Joseph E. Ransdell to Charles Holmes Herty, December 19, 1928, Herty Papers, Box 103, folder 9. Harvey W. Wiley's article, published in the March 1929 *Good Housekeeping*, urged readers to contact their congressmen on behalf of the bill in order to "do your part in protecting the health of your own children and the children of the future." See the reprinted article in U.S. Congress, Senate, *Congressional Record*, 70th Cong., 2nd sess., March 1, 1929, pp. 4822–23; quotation is from p. 4823.

30. PHS *Annual Report*, 1929, p. 4.

31. "Influenza Cases Mount to 700,000," *New York Times*, December 20, 1928, p. 15.

32. Royal S. Copeland to Joseph E. Ransdell, January 3, 1929, Herty Papers, Box 104, folder 1. Although primarily a supporter of Ransdell in the effort to establish a National Institute of Health, Copeland later became the sponsor and champion of the bill that became the Food, Drug, and Cosmetic Act of 1938. See Young, *The Medical Messiahs*, pp. 164–90; Charles O. Jackson, *Food and Drug Legislation in the New Deal* (Princeton: Princeton University Press, 1970).

33. Ransdell to Charles Holmes Herty, January 5, 1928, Herty Papers Box 104, folder 1.

34. Fullaway to H. M. Lord, January 15, 1929, File "S. 4540, 69th Cong., NIH," Box 265, Series 21.2, Budget Bureau, Treasury Department Records, RG 51, NA.

35. Cumming to Charles Holmes Herty, February 5, 1929, Herty Papers, Box 104, folder 1.

36. Andrew Mellon to Wesley L. Jones, January 21, 1929, Herty Papers, Box 104, folder 1. Ransdell also had the letter entered in the *Congressional Record*, 70th Cong., 2nd sess., February 6, 1929, p. 2914.

37. Herty to Joseph E. Ransdell, January 7, 1929, Herty Papers, Box 104, folder 1.

38. Ransdell to Charles Holmes Herty, January 25, 1929, Herty Papers, Box 104, folder 1.

39. U.S. Congress, Senate, *Congressional Record*, 70th Cong., 2nd sess., January 24, 1929, p. 2160.

40. Ibid.

41. Telegram, Joseph E. Ransdell to Charles Holmes Herty, January 25, 1929, Herty Papers, Box 104, folder 1.

42. "Team Work of Science," *New York Times*, January 27, 1929, III, p. 4.

43. Herty to Joseph E. Ransdell, January 29, 1929, Herty Papers, Box 104, folder 1.

44. U.S. Congress, Senate, *Congressional Record*, 70th Cong., 2nd sess., February 6, 1929, pp. 2905–10.

45. Ibid., pp. 2911, 2913.

46. Ibid., p. 2193.

47. Ransdell to Charles Holmes Herty, February 7, 1929, Herty Papers, Box 104, folder 1.

48. Herty to Joseph E. Ransdell, February 13, 1929, Herty Papers, Box 104, folder 1.

49. Herty to Armistead Holcombe, February 15, 1929, Herty Papers, Box 104, folder 1.

50. "The Nation's Health," *New York Times*, February 20, 1929, p. 24.

51. Ransdell to Charles Holmes Herty, February 15, 1929, Herty Papers, Box 104, folder 1.

52. Ibid.

53. Herty to Joseph E. Ransdell, February 13, 1929, Herty Papers, Box 104, folder 1.

54. Ransdell to Charles Holmes Herty, March 9, 1929, Herty Papers, Box 104, folder 2. The text of the revised bill is recorded in U.S. Congress, Senate, *Congressional Record*, 70th Cong., 2nd sess., March 1, 1929, p. 4891.

55. Ibid.

56. Ibid.

57. U.S. Congress, House, *Congressional Record*, 70th Cong., 2nd sess., March 3, 1929, p. 5204.

58. Ibid., p. 5206.

59. Ibid., pp. 5204, 5206.

60. Herty to Franklin Hobbs, April 1, 1929, Herty Papers, Box 104, folder 2.

61. Ibid.

62. Herty to Francis Garvan, March 19, 1929, Herty Papers, Box 104, folder 4.

63. Herty to Joseph E. Ransdell, April 8, 1929, Herty Papers, Box 104, folder 2.

64. Ransdell to Charles Holmes Herty, March 9, 1929, Herty Papers, Box 104, folder 2. Herty believed that Congressman Sirovich should not handle the legislation again "because of prejudice against him, and his failure to do anything about" the Ransdell bill "after he had introduced it." Sirovich, although a surgeon, was Jewish and opposed to prohibition. These characteristics may explain the "prejudice" Herty noted. See Herty to Franklin Hobbs, April 1, 1929, Herty Papers, Box 104, folder 2; U.S. Congress, House, *Biographical Directory of the American Congress*, pp. 1702–3.

65. George W. McCoy, Memorandum on Bills to Provide a National Institute of Health, March 16, 1929, File OD, .0221, NIH, PHS Records, RG 90, NA.

66. Ibid.

67. Ransdell to Charles Holmes Herty, April 22, 1929, Herty Papers, Box 104, folder 2.

68. Herty to James S. Parker, April 23, 1929, Herty Papers, Box 104, folder 2; Ransdell to Charles Holmes Herty, May 4, 1929, Herty Papers, Box 104, folder 3.

69. Ransdell to Charles Holmes Herty, May 4, 1929; clipping from *U.S. Daily*, May 4, 1929, Herty Papers, Box 104, folder 3.

70. Ransdell to Charles Holmes Herty, May 7, 1929, Herty Papers, Box 104, folder 3.

71. Ray Lyman Wilbur to Joseph E. Ransdell, May 9, 1929, Herty Papers, Box 104, folder 3.

72. Ransdell to James S. Parker, May 11, 1929, Herty Papers, Box 104, folder 3.

73. U.S. Congress, Senate, *A Bill to Establish and Operate a National Institute of Health, to Create A System of Fellowships in Said Institute, and to Authorize the Government to Accept Donations for Use in Ascertaining the Cause, Prevention, and Cure of Disease Affecting Human Beings, and for Other Purposes*, S. 1171, 71st Cong., 1st sess., May 20, 1929. A copy of the bill is in the Herty Papers, Box 104, folder 9.

74. Memorandum, Charles H. Fullaway to R. O. Kloeber, June 1, 1929, File "S. 4540, 69th Cong., NIH," Box 265, Series 21.2, Budget Bureau, Treasury Department Records, RG 51, NA.

75. Mellon to Wesley L. Jones, July 25, 1929, Herty Papers, Box 104, folder 3.

76. Ransdell to Charles Holmes Herty, August 16, 1929, Herty Papers, Box 104, folder 3.

77. U.S. Congress, House, *A Bill to Provide for the Coordination of the*

Public Health Activities of the Government and for Other Purposes, H.R. 3142, 71st Cong., 1st sess., May 20, 1929. A copy of the bill is in File 1220 General, PHS General Subject Files, 1924–35; also in notebook four, "1929–1930," Coordination Notebooks; PHS Records, RG 90, NA. An identical form of this bill was introduced into the Senate as S. 1195 by the chairman of the Commerce Committee, Wesley Jones.

78. One minor addition to section one stipulated that detailed officers would be paid out of Public Health Service funds.

79. The Service prepared a side-by-side comparison of the old and new versions of the bill. Throughout are references to the deletion of unconstitutional language. See File 1220 General, PHS General Subject Files, 1924–35, PHS Records, RG 90, NA.

80. Ibid.

81. *An Act to Establish Two United States Narcotic Farms for the Confinement and Treatment of Persons Addicted to the Use of Habit-Forming Narcotic Drugs Who Have Been Convicted of Offenses against the United States, and for Other Purposes*, Act of January 19, 1929, 45 *Stat. L.* 1085.

82. Side-by-side comparison of versions of Parker bill, File 1220 General, PHS General Subject Files, 1924–35, PHS Records, RG 90, NA.

83. Williams, *USPHS*, pp. 547–49.

84. U.S. Congress, S. Rept. 101 to Accompany S. 3167, 71st Cong., 2nd sess., January 18, 1930, p. 6; Furman, *Profile*, p. 287; Miles, "Further Development of the Public Health Service by the Parker Act, 1930," p. 19.

85. Cumming to John D. Long, January 30, 1929, Cumming Papers, AN 6922, Box 17, folder 5.

86. Ibid.

87. Cumming to F. C. Warnshuis, December 12, 1929, Cumming Papers, AN 6922, Box 17, folder 3.

88. Hugh S. Cumming autobiography, p. 382, Cumming Papers, AN 6922-K.

89. Cumming to William H. Welch, September 3, 1929, File 1220 General, PHS General Files, 1924–35, PHS Records, RG 90, NA.

90. J. Clawson Roop to Treasury Secretary Andrew Mellon, December 20, 1929, notebook four, "1929–1930," Coordination Notebooks, PHS Records, RG 90, NA.

91. Cumming to J. D. Long, January 28, 1930, Cumming Papers, AN 6922, Box 18, folder 3.

92. J. Clawson Roop to Treasury Secretary Andrew Mellon, January 10, 1930, notebook four, "1929–1930," Coordination Notebooks, PHS Records, RG 90, NA.

93. U.S. Congress, House Rept. 542 to Accompany H.R. 8807, 71st Cong., 2nd sess., January 28, 1930; S. Rept. 101 to Accompany S. 3167, 71st Cong., 2nd sess., January 18, 1930.

94. Herty to James S. Parker, December 12, 1929, Herty Papers, Box 104, folder 3.

95. Herty to James S. Parker, December 19, 1929, Herty Papers, Box 104, folder 3.

96. James S. Parker to Charles Holmes Herty, December 20, 1929, Herty Papers, Box 104, folder 3.

97. Ransdell to Charles Holmes Herty, January 18, 1930, Herty Papers, Box 104, folder 4.

98. H. B. Anderson to Nicholas Longworth, February 3, 1930, Herty Papers, Box 104, folder 4; "The Public Health Service: One Finds Senator Ransdell's Bill Raises Numerous Questions," letter to the editor from H. B. Anderson, *New York Times*, February 25, 1929, p. 22

99. Herty to Mildred E. Reeves, February 13, 1930, Herty Papers, Box 104, folder 4.

100. Cumming to Francis D. Patterson, March 17, 1930, Cumming Papers, AN 6922, Box 18, folder 3.

101. For a discussion of the psittacosis epidemic see Williams, *USPHS*, pp. 215–18; Furman, *Profile*, pp. 370–73. A popular account is in De Kruif, *Men Against Death*, ch. 6.

102. Cumming to Thomas Parran, March 17, 1930, Cumming Papers, AN 6922, Box 18, folder 3.

103. U.S. Congress, House, *Congressional Record*, 71st Cong., 2nd sess., March 26, 1930, p. 6121.

104. Ibid., p. 6122.

105. Ibid., p. 6124.

106. Two minor amendments were also approved with this vote. The first was a one word grammatical correction; the second, a stipulation offered by Congressman Crosser that in the appointment of Service employees no preference would be given to any school of medicine.

107. Ransdell to Charles Holmes Herty, March 24, 1930, Herty Papers, Box 104, folder 4.

108. Telegram, Lee Wilson to Joseph E. Ransdell, April 1, 1930; telegram, Lois Woodford to Charles Holmes Herty, April 1, 1930, Herty Papers, Box 104, folder 4. The bill's passage is recorded in U.S. Congress, Senate, *Congressional Record*, 71st Cong., 2nd sess., April 1, 1930, p. 6252.

109. Hugh S. Cumming autobiography, p. 388, Cumming Papers, AN 6922-K.

110. Ibid.

111. U.S. Congress, Senate, *Congressional Record*, 71st Cong., 2nd sess., April 1, 1930, p. 6252. The approved amendment deleted the section of the bill that created two senior Medical Directors.

112. U.S., Congress, House, *Congressional Record*, 71st Cong., 2nd sess., April 2, 1930, p. 6394; *An Act to Provide for the Coordination of the Public Health Activities of the Government, and for Other Purposes*, 71st Cong., 2nd sess., April 9, 1930, P.L. 71-106, 46 *Stat. L.* 150.

113. See correspondence throughout April 1930, Cumming Papers, AN 6922, Box 18, folder 4.

114. Cumming to Lee K. Frankel, April 21, 1930, Cumming Papers, AN 6922, Box 18, folder 4.

115. Cumming to Rupert Blue, April 22, 1930, Cumming Papers, AN 6922, Box 18, folder 4.

116. Mildred E. Reeves to Charles Holmes Herty, April 3, 1930, Herty Papers, Box 104, folder 4.

117. Ransdell to Charles Holmes Herty, April 12, 1930, Herty Papers, Box 104, folder 4.

118. Herty to John H. Finley, April 26, 1930, Herty Papers, Box 104, folder 4; "The Last Enemy," *New York Times*, April 21, 1930, p. 22.

119. U.S. Congress, House Committee on Interstate and Foreign Commerce, *National Institute of Health: Hearing Before the Committee on Interstate and Foreign Commerce on S. 1171*, 71st Cong., 2nd sess., April 21, 1930, pp. 7, 16.

120. Ibid., p. 2.

121. Ibid., p. 18.

122. Ibid.

123. Ibid., p. 8.

124. Ibid., pp. 12, 13.

125. Ibid., pp. 24–32.

126. Ibid., pp. 26, 28.

127. Ransdell to Andrew Mellon, May 5, 1930, File OD, .0221, NIH, PHS Records, RG 90, NA.

128. U.S. Congress, House Rept. 1461 to Accompany S. 1171, 71st Cong., 2nd sess., May 15, 1930; *Congressional Record*, 71st Cong., 2nd sess., May 19, 1930, p. 9180.

129. Telegram, Joseph E. Ransdell to Charles Holmes Herty, May 14, 1930, Herty Papers, Box 104, folder 4.

130. U.S. Congress, House, *Congressional Record*, 71st Cong., 2nd sess., May 19, 1930, p. 9182.

131. Ibid.

132. Ibid., p. 9181.

133. Ibid.

134. Ibid., p. 9183.

135. U.S. Congress, Senate, *Congressional Record*, 71st Cong., 2nd sess., May 21, 1930, p. 9259.

136. "Hoover Signs Health Bill," *New York Times*, May 27, 1930, p. 29; *An Act to Establish and Operate a National Institute of Health, to Create a System of Fellowships in Said Institute, and to Authorize the Government to Accept Donations for Use in Ascertaining the Cause, Prevention, and Cure of Disease Affecting Human Beings, and for Other Purposes*, 71st Cong., 2nd sess., May 26, 1930, P.L. 71-251, 46 *Stat. L.* 379.

137. U.S. Congress, Senate, *Congressional Record*, 71st Cong., 2nd sess., May 21, 1930, p. 9259.

Eight: A National Institute of Health

1. Charles Holmes Herty to committee members, May 27, 1930, Herty Papers, Box 104, folder 4.

2. Herty to the president of the American Chemical Society, March 9, 1931, Herty Papers, Box 102, folder 10.

3. "A New Health Institute," *New York Times*, May 24, 1930, p. 16.

4. *How to Conserve Public Health—The Most Important Problem Confronting Mankind: The National Institute of Health: Remarks of the Hon. Joseph E. Ransdell, the Hon. Royal S. Copeland, and the Hon. Henry D. Hatfield, in the Senate of the United States, February 26, 1931* (Washington, D.C.: Government Printing Office, 1931).

5. Conference Board of the National Institute of Health, U.S. Public Health Service, Summarized Report for the Year Beginning March 18, 1931 and Ending March 18, 1932, pp. 1–2, Herty Papers, Box 104, folder 6. Hereafter cited as Conference Board Summarized Report, 1931–32.

6. U.S. Congress, Senate, *Congressional Record*, 71st Cong., 2nd sess., June 10, 1930, pp. 10358–62; U.S. Congress, House, *Congressional Record*, 71st Cong., 2nd sess., June 16, 1930, pp. 10951–53.

7. Hudson Grunewald, "War Declared on Disease—Capital to be Center of Biggest Fight Ever Waged under Plans Approved by Congress," *Washington Star*, June 15, 1930, reprinted in U.S., Congress, House, *Congressional Record*, 71st Cong., 2nd sess., June 16, 1930, p. 10951.

8. Francis Garvan to Joseph E. Ransdell, June 20, 1930, reprinted in U.S. Congress, Senate, *Congressional Record*, 71st Cong., 2nd sess., June 23, 1930, p. 11501.

9. Joseph E. Ransdell to Francis Garvan, June 23, 1930, reprinted in U.S. Congress, Senate, *Congressional Record*, 71st Cong., 2nd sess., June 23, 1930, p. 11501.

10. Ransdell to Herbert Hoover, draft of letter, n.d., Box 2, folder 13, Joseph E. Ransdell Papers, Department of Archives, Middleton Library, Louisiana State University, Baton Rouge. Hereafter cited as Ransdell Papers.

11. Ransdell to Herbert Hoover, December 30, 1930, Letter quoted within another letter, Ransdell to Hoover, March 31, 1931, Cumming Papers, AN 6922, Box 20, folder 1.

12. Ransdell to Herbert Hoover, March 31, 1931, Cumming Papers, AN 6922, Box 20, folder 1.

13. Ibid.

14. Ransdell to Hugh S. Cumming, March 30, 1931, Cumming Papers, AN 6922, Box 20, folder 1.

15. Minutes of the Organizational Meeting of the Conference Board of the National Institute of Health, March 18, 1931, Cumming Papers, AN 6922, Box 20, folder 1.

16. Conference Board Summarized Report, 1931–32, p. 1, Herty Papers, Box 104, folder 6.

17. Minutes of the Organizational Meeting of the Conference Board of the National Institute of Health, March 18, 1931, Cumming Papers, AN 6922, Box 20, folder 1.

18. Conference Board Summarized Report, 1931–32, p. 1, Herty Papers, Box 104, folder 6.

19. Ibid., pp. 1–2.

20. Conference Board of the National Institute of Health, U.S. Public Health

Service, Fourth Quarterly Report, March 18, 1932, p. 2, Herty Papers, Box 104, folder 6; Synopsis of Address Delivered by Former Senator Jos. E. Ransdell of Louisiana before a Meeting of the Parent-Teacher's Association of Washington, D.C., Tuesday Evening, April 21, 1931, 6:30 p.m., Herty Papers, Box 104, folder 5.

21. Conference Board of the National Institute of Health, U.S. Public Health Service, Fourth Quarterly Report, March 18, 1932, p. 2; Quarterly Report of the Executive Director, Conference Board of the National Institute of Health, September 18, 1932, p. 1; Quarterly Report of the Executive Director, Conference Board of the National Institute of Health, December 19, 1932, p. 2, Herty Papers, Box 104, folder 6.

22. Report of Jos. E. Ransdell, Executive Director of the Conference Board of the National Institute of Health, July 31, 1933, p. 2, Herty Papers, Box 104, folder 6.

23. Conference Board Summarized Report, 1931–32, p. 2, Herty Papers, Box 104, folder 6. The contribution of the Conference Board was the amount Ransdell received from *Commonweal* for an article he wrote about the Institute.

24. Quarterly Report of the Executive Director, Conference Board of the National Institute of Health, June 20, 1932, p. 1, Herty Papers, Box 104, folder 6.

25. Third Quarterly Report of the Executive Director of the Conference Board of the National Institute of Health, December 18, 1931, p. 1, Herty Papers, Box 104, folder 5.

26. Quarterly Report of the Executive Director, Conference Board of the National Institute of Health, June 2, 1932, p. 1, Herty Papers, Box 104, folder 6.

27. Ibid.

28. Quarterly Report of the Executive Director, Conference Board of the National Institute of Health, September 18, 1932, p. 1, Herty Papers, Box 104, folder 6.

29. Ibid.

30. Ibid.

31. Report of Jos. E. Ransdell, Executive Director of the Conference Board of the National Institute of Health, July 31, 1933, p. 3, Herty Papers, Box 104, folder 6.

32. John A. Garraty, *The American Nation*, 2nd ed. (New York: Harper & Row, 1971), pp. 828–35.

33. Ransdell to Edgar B. Rickard of the A.R.A. Children's Fund, January 21, 1933, Ransdell Papers, Box 2, folder 4.

34. Preliminary Plan for the National Health Foundation, February 9, 1933, Herty Papers, Box 104, folder 6.

35. J. C. Funk to Joseph E. Ransdell, May 31, 1933, Ransdell Papers, Box 2, folder 11.

36. See Statement on the National Health Foundation with list of board of trustees attached to letter from Ransdell to Charles Holmes Herty, February 9, 1933, Herty Papers, Box 104, folder 4.

37. Joseph Colt Bloodgood to Joseph E. Ransdell, March 29, 1933, Ransdell Papers, Box 2, folder 4.

38. Ransdell to H. Edmund Bullis, April 4, 1933, Ransdell Papers, Box 2, folder 4.

39. Ibid.

40. See correspondence and information on the National Health Foundation in Ransdell Papers, Box 2, folder 4; Herty Papers, Box 104, folder 6.

41. Ransdell to Charles Holmes Herty, July 17, 1933, Herty Papers, Box 104, folder 6.

42. Grunewald, "War Declared on Disease," *Washington Star*, reprinted in *Congressional Record*, p. 10953.

43. La Borde, *National Southerner*, pp. 179–80.

44. Thomas Parran to Joseph E. Ransdell, May 20, 1938, Ransdell Papers, Box 3, folder 21.

45. Joseph W. Montgomery to Joseph E. Ransdell, June 6, 1938, Ransdell Papers, Box 3, folder 21.

46. "A Crusader," pp. 963–64.

47. Morey, "Charles Holmes Herty," pp. 1441–42.

48. Meeting of the National Advisory Health Council, April 9 and 10, 1931, p. 1, Box 34, File 0240-12, "National Advisory Health Council, 1925–1935," PHS General Subject Files, 1924–35, PHS Records, RG 90, NA. Hereafter cited as File 0240-12, "NAHC, 1925–1935."

49. Ibid., p. 4.

50. Ibid., pp. 5–7.

51. Ibid., pp. 3–4.

52. Hugh S. Cumming to Francis Garvan, September 13, 1932; Cumming to Garvan, August 19, 1935, Box 170, File 150, "Chemical Foundation," PHS General Subject Files, 1924–35, PHS Records, RG 90, NA; PHS *Annual Report*, 1932, pp. 71–72; 1933, p. 38; 1934, pp. 40–41; 1935, p. 53; 1936, p. 50. Purves's research was published in a series of articles, many with Claude S. Hudson, entitled "Analysis of Fructoside Mixtures by Means of Invertase," *Journal of the American Chemical Society* 56: 702–7, 56: 708–11, 56: 1969–73, 56: 1973–77 (1934); 59: 49–56, 59: 1170–74 (1937).

53. Meeting of the National Advisory Health Council, April 9 and 10, 1931, p. 7, File 0240-12, "NAHC, 1925–1935," PHS General Subject Files, 1924–35, PHS Records, RG 90, NA.

54. Ibid., p. 8.

55. Ibid., pp. 8–10.

56. Ibid., p. 8.

57. Ibid., p. 12.

58. Ibid., pp. 14–15.

59. Ibid., p. 12.

60. Ibid., p. 13.

61. *Notable Contributions*, p. 41; Meeting of the National Advisory Health Council, April 9 and 10, 1931, p. 14, File 0240-12, "NAHC 1925–1935," PHS General Subject Files, 1924–35, PHS Records, RG 90, NA.

62. Meeting of the National Advisory Health Council, April 9 and 10, 1931,

pp. 13–14, File 0240-12, "NAHC, 1925–1935," PHS General Subject Files, 1924–35, PHS Records, RG 90, NA.

63. Cumming to Undersecretary and Budget Officer, Treasury Department, April 17, 1933, File "Federal Government Reorganization—Recommendations of 1933—General Correspondence," Parran Papers.

64. Ibid. Cumming wrote several letters and memoranda to the Budget Officer on different subjects, all of which are dated April 17, 1933. The letter cited here is a separate one from the one cited in note 63.

65. For biographical information on McCoy see Clark, *Pioneer Microbiologists of America*, p. 212; Charles Armstrong, unpublished biography of McCoy, 1960, National Library of Medicine; Williams, *USPHS*, pp. 252–53.

66. Armstrong, unpublished biography, p. 12.

67. Ibid., pp. 9–12; Victor H. Kramer, *The National Institute of Health: A Study in Public Administration* (New Haven: Quinnipiack Press, 1937), pp. 13, 22–23, 67–68.

68. Kramer, *National Institute of Health*, p. 68.

69. Ibid.

70. Ibid.

71. For a discussion of McCoy's departure from the Institute, see Furman, *Profile*, pp. 397–98.

72. Michael B. Shimkin, interview with author, March 17, 1982.

73. For biographical information on Parran see File "Parran—Biographical Data," Parran Papers; Williams, *USPHS*, pp. 484–86; obituaries in *JAMA* 203: 36 (March 11, 1968); *AJPH* 58: 615–17 (April 1968); *New York Times*, February 17, 1968, pp. 1, 29.

74. Parran to Alice Kinyoun (Mrs. Hale) Houts, n.d., File "Miscellaneous Bibliography," Parran Papers.

75. Michael B. Shimkin, interview with author, March 17, 1982. See also Shimkin's comments on Parran as Surgeon General in his *As Memory Serves: Six Essays on a Personal Involvement with the National Cancer Institute, 1938 to 1978* (Washington, D.C.: National Institutes of Health, NIH Publication No. 83-2217, 1983), p. 10.

76. Bess Furman, interview with Thomas Parran, p. 4, Box 7, notebook 1, "Dr. Parran Section," in Bess Furman Armstrong, Materials Pertaining to the History of the Public Health Service, National Library of Medicine.

77. For biographical information on Thompson see Williams, *USPHS*, pp. 253–54; obituaries in *JAMA* 157: 160 (January 8, 1955); *New York Times*, November 14, 1954, p. 88.

78. L. R. Thompson to Thomas Parran, August 18, 1933, File "Federal Government Reorganization—Recommendations of 1933—General Correspondence," Parran Papers.

79. Parran to C.-E. A. Winslow, May 15, 1933, File "Federal Government Reorganization—Recommendations of 1933—General Correspondence," Parran Papers.

80. Parran, "Reorganization of Federal Health Services," Memorandum and three charts showing existing organization, reorganization proposed by Herbert Hoover, and "a plan for more complete reorganization," January 18,

1933, File "Federal Government Reorganization—Recommendations of 1933—General Correspondence," Parran Papers.

81. *NIH Almanac*, 1981, pp. 5–6.

82. Cumming to J. W. Kerr, July 8, 1930, File "National Institute of Health—Correspondence, 1930–1935," Parran Papers.

83. Cumming to Atherton Seidell, August 7, 1930, Cumming Papers, AN 6922, Box 18, folder 4.

84. Parran to L. R. Thompson, September 11, 1930, File "National Institute of Health—Correspondence, 1930–1935," Parran Papers.

85. Don S. Warran, "New Buildings Here to Intensify War on Disease," *Washington Evening Star*, August 30, 1932, Building Section, p. 1.

86. L. R. Thompson, "Development of the National Institute of Health from 1930–1938," National Institute of Health, Copies of Documents Placed in Cornerstone of Building 1 at NIH Dedication in 1938, National Library of Medicine.

87. Ibid.; Furman, *Profile*, p. 397; Michael B. Shimkin, interview with author, March 17, 1982.

88. L. R. Thompson, "Development of the National Institute of Health from 1930–1938."

89. My discussion of this episode follows that of Donald C. Swain in his article, "The Rise of a Research Empire: NIH, 1930–1950," *Science* 138: 1233–37 (December 14, 1962); quotation is from p. 1234.

90. PHS *Annual Report*, 1931, p. 10.

91. Ibid., 1932, p. 43.

92. Ibid., 1931, p. 11.

93. Ibid.

94. Ibid., 1938, p. 63.

95. Ibid., 1932, p. 25.

96. Ibid., 1931, pp. 9–10; 1932, pp. 22–25; 1933, pp. 17–19; 1934, pp. 15–18.

97. On the creation of the National Cancer Institute see Wyndham Miles, "Creation of National Cancer Institute," unpublished manuscript, n.d., National Library of Medicine; J. R. Heller, "The National Cancer Institute: A Twenty Year Retrospect," *Journal of the National Cancer Institute* 19: 147–90 (1957); Strickland, *Politics, Science, and Dread Disease*, pp. 1–14.

98. Swain, "Rise of a Research Empire," pp. 1234–35.

99. *An Act to Consolidate and Revise the Laws Relating to the Public Health Service, and for Other Purposes*, July 1, 1944, 58 *Stat. L.* 682.

100. Ibid.

Epilogue: A Century of Science for Health

1. For surveys dealing with postwar developments see Swain, "Rise of a Research Empire;" Strickland, *Politics, Science, and Dread Disease*; G. Burroughs Mider, "The Federal Impact on Biomedical Research," in Bowers and Purcell, eds., *Advances in American Medicine*, 2: 806–71; James A. Shannon, "The Advancement of Medical Research: A Twenty-Year View of the Role

of the National Institutes of Health," *Journal of Medical Education* 42: 97–108 (February 1967); Donald S. Fredrickson, "The National Institutes of Health Yesterday, Today, and Tomorrow," *Public Health Reports* 93: 642–47 (November-December 1978); Elizabeth Brenner Drew, "The Health Syndicate: Washington's Noble Conspirators," *Atlantic Monthly* 220: 75–82 (December 1967); Natalie Davis Spingarn, *Heartbeat: The Politics of Health Research* (Washington, D.C.: Robert B. Luce, 1976).

2. Vannevar Bush, *Science—The Endless Frontier: A Report to the President* (Washington, D.C.: Government Printing Office, 1945). For the history of the writing of this report see England, *A Patron for Pure Science*, pp. 9–23.

3. U.S. President's Scientific Research Board, *Science and Public Policy: A Report to the President* by John R. Steelman, 5 vols. (Washington, D.C.: Government Printing Office, 1947). Definitions of the different types of research are in vol. 5, *The Nation's Medical Research*, p. 8.

4. Comments on the development of this decision by a member of the Steelman committee are in an interview with Norman H. Topping, in George Rosen, "Transcripts of Oral History project, 1962–1964," History of Medicine Division, National Library of Medicine, pp. 31–35.

5. *NIH Almanac*, 1983, pp. 6, 8.

6. Swain, "Rise of a Research Empire," pp. 1235–36.

7. *NIH Almanac*, 1983, p. 5.

8. Young, "Public Policy and Drug Innovation," pp. 8–9; John Parascandola, ed., *The History of Antibiotics: A Symposium* (Madison, Wis.: American Institute of the History of Pharmacy, 1980); Dowling, *Fighting Infection*, pp. 125–57; A. N. Richards, "Production of Penicillin in the United States (1941–1946)," *Nature* 201: 441–45 (1964); Selman A. Waksman, "The Microbiology of the Soil and the Antibiotics," in Iago Galdston, ed., *The Impact of the Antibiotics on Medicine and Society* (New York: International Universities Press, 1958), pp. 3–7.

9. A. N. Richards, "The Impact of the War on Medicine," *Science* 103: 578 (May 10, 1946); Young, "Public Policy and Drug Innovation," p. 8; James A. Shannon, "Chemotherapy in Malaria," *Bulletin of the New York Academy of Medicine* 22: 345–57 (1946); G. R. Coatney, "Pitfalls in a Discovery: The Chronicle of Chloroquine," *American Journal of Tropical Medicine and Hygiene* 12: 121–28 (1963); Harry F. Dowling, *Medicines for Man* (New York: Alfred A. Knopf, 1970), pp. 19, 36–37; Irvin Stewart, *Organizing Scientific Research for War* (Boston: Little, Brown & Co,, 1948); E. C. Andrus et al., eds., *Advances in Military Medicine Made by American Investigators Working under the Sponsorship of the Committee on Medical Research* (Boston: Little, Brown & Co., 1948).

10. Young, "Public Policy and Drug Innovation," pp. 9–10; on confronting peacetime urgencies with wartime problem-solving methods, see William E. Leuchtenburg, "The New Deal and the Analogue of War," in John Braemer, Robert H. Bremner and Everett Walters, eds., *Change and Continuity in Twentieth-Century America* (Columbus: Ohio State University Press, 1964); on the "fight on cancer" see Clarence Cook Little, *The Fight on Cancer* (New York: Public Affairs Committee, 1939).

11. Strickland discusses these developments at length; see *Politics, Science, and Dread Disease*, pp. 55–133.

12. Ibid., pp. 134–83; see also James B. Wyngaarden, "Nurturing the Scientific Enterprise," *Journal of Medical Education* 59: 155 (March 1984).

13. Biographical information on Shannon is in Jaques Cattell Press, ed., *American Men and Women of Science*, 15th ed., *Physical and Biological Sciences*, 7 vols. (New York: R. R. Bowker Co., 1982), 6: 628; *NIH Almanac*, 1983, p. 121.

14. Figures are from the *NIH Almanac*, 1983, p. 121 and from NIH budget figures, 1950–84, Division of Financial Management, National Institutes of Health.

15. *NIH Almanac*, 1983, p. 134. For an evaluation of the contribution of NIH grants to the development of biomedical research in other countries see Sune Bergström, "American Support of International Biomedical Research Programs: A Swedish Viewpoint," in Bowers and Purcell, eds., *Advances in American Medicine*, 2: 789–805.

16. *NIH Almanac*, 1983, pp. 168–70. The research of the four NIH intramural Nobel laureates is described in De Witt Stetten, Jr. and W. T. Carrigan, eds., *NIH: An Account of Research in Its Laboratories and Clinics* (New York: Academic Press, 1984): Marshall Nirenberg (1968 Nobel prize for "Physiology or Medicine," shared with two other scientists), pp. 285–300; Julius Axelrod (1970 Nobel prize for "Physiology or Medicine," shared with two other scientists), pp. 30–32, 40–45; Christian B. Anfinsen (1972 Nobel prize for "Chemistry," shared with two other scientists), pp. 259–65; D. Carleton Gajdusek (1976 Nobel prize for "Physiology or Medicine," shared with one other scientist), pp. 395–415.

17. Harold M. Schmeck, Jr., "Research Called Crucial in Health," *New York Times*, July 19, 1968, p. 23.

18. "Early Detection of Uterine Cancer," U.S. Department of Health, Education & Welfare, Public Health Service, National Institutes of Health, *Progress Reports* 19: 1–4 (November 1954). Hereafter cited as *Progress Reports* (NIH). A concise list of such NIH contributions is in "Highlights in the History and Organization of the National Institutes of Health, 1945–1975," in-house booklet, National Institutes of Health, n.d.

19. "The New Oral Antidiabetic Drugs," *Progress Reports* (NIH) 64: 1–4 (December 1956).

20. "Surgical Treatment of Congenital Heart Disease," *Progress Reports* (NIH) 35: 1–5 (January 1955).

21. "Highlights of Progress in Research on Allergy and Infectious Diseases, 1960," in *Research Highlights: National Institutes of Health, 1960: Items of Interest on Program Developments and Research Studies Conducted and Supported by the Institutes and Divisions of NIH as Presented to the Congress of the United States* (Washington, D.C.: U.S. Department of Health, Education & Welfare, 1960), pp. 97–99.

22. Starr, *Social Transformation of American Medicine*, pp. 335–419.

23. D. S. Greenberg, "NIH: As the Time Approaches for Shannon's Retirement," *Science* 158: 1166 (December 1, 1967).

24. "An Overview of the National High Blood Pressure Education Program," in-house document prepared for the Senate Blue Ribbon Committee for Evaluation of the National High Blood Pressure Education Program, September 1979, National Heart, Lung, and Blood Institute.

25. On the history of the National Library of Medicine see Wyndham Miles, *A History of the National Library of Medicine: The Nation's Treasury of Medical Knowledge* (Washington, D.C.: U.S. Department of Health and Human Services, Publication No. (NIH) 82-1904), especially pp. 343–91; 411–41.

26. At this time, 400 institutions in the United States received a quarter of a billion dollars to support 11,500 research projects. Of these institutions, however, 200 received 90 percent of all monies awarded. See Strickland, *Politics, Science, and Dread Disease*, pp. 169–70.

27. Robert S. Stone, "Care and Feeding of Excellence—The Science Administrator's Raison d'etre," Speech presented at Brooklyn College, New York, January 24, 1974, in National Institutes of Health (U.S.), Office of the Director, "Speeches and Articles of Dr. Robert S. Stone," unpublished manuscript, n.d., National Institutes of Health Library, Bethesda, Md., n.p.

28. Donald S. Fredrickson, "Research and the Political Process," Speech to the Federation of American Societies for Experimental Biology, April 4, 1977, Chicago, in National Institutes of Health (U.S.), Office of the Director, "Speeches, Articles, and Selected Papers of Donald S. Fredrickson, 1975–1981," 3 vols., unpublished manuscript, n.d., National Institutes of Health Library, Bethesda, Md., 2: document 49, pp. 4–5.

29. An expansion of the initiative begun in 1955, for example, screened by 1976 over four hundred thousand synthetic and natural products for their usefulness in treating cancer. See Young, "Public Policy and Drug Innovation," p. 10. On the "War on Cancer" see "The National Cancer Act of 1971," *Journal of the National Cancer Institute* 48: 577–84 (March 1972); Richard A. Rettig, *Cancer Crusade: The Story of the National Cancer Act of 1971* (Princeton: Princeton University Press, 1977).

30. Irvine H. Page, "Another Crusade!" *Science* 176: 967 (June 2, 1972).

31. Max Tishler, "The Public Stake in Medical Research," *Proceedings of the Royal Society of Medicine* 61: 691–93 (1968), cited in Young, "Public Policy and Drug Innovation," p. 10, note 45.

32. Barbara J. Culliton, "Health Hierarchy: Marston Fired and He's Not the Only One," *Science* 178: 1268–70 (December 22, 1972); Culliton, "Back at NIH, Marston's Firing Prompts Mild Protest," *Science* 179: 260–61 (January 19, 1973).

33. Barbara J. Culliton, "NIH: Robert Stone Is in Trouble with HEW," *Science* 186: 615–17, 667 (November 15, 1974).

34. Barbara J. Culliton, "NIH Advisory Committees: The Politics of Filling Vacancies," *Science* 190: 443–44 (October 31, 1975).

35. Sherwin and Isenson, *First Interim Report on Project Hindsight*.

36. David Schwartzman, *Innovation in the Pharmaceutical Industry* (Baltimore: Johns Hopkins University Press, 1976). My discussion of Schwartzman's ideas is taken from Young, "Public Policy and Drug Innovation," p. 18.

37. Fredrickson, "Research and the Political Process," pp. 3–9.

38. Barbara J. Culliton, "FAS Attacks Politicization of NIH," *Science* 187: 47 (January 10, 1975).

39. Ivan L. Bennett, Jr., "Application of Biomedical Knowledge: The White House View," in *Research in the Service of Man*, p. 9.

40. J. H. Comroe and R. D. Dripps, "Ben Franklin and Open-Heart Surgery," *Circulation Research* 35: 661–69 (November 1974); other articles on this subject are Comroe, "Lags Between Initial Discovery and Clinical Application to Cardiovascular Pulmonary Medicine and Surgery," *Report of the President's Biomedical Research Panel* (Washington, D.C.: U.S. Department of Health, Education & Welfare, DHEW Publication No. (OS) 76-502), Appendix B; Comroe and Dripps, "Scientific Basis for the Support of Biomedical Sciences."

41. James B. Wyngaarden, "Directions and Challenges in Health Sciences Research," *Environmental Health Perspectives* 52: 274 (1983).

42. National Academy of Sciences, Institute of Medicine, Division of Health Sciences Policy, *Responding to Health Needs and Scientific Opportunity: The Organizational Structure of the National Institutes of Health* (Washington, D.C.: National Academy Press, 1984), p. 37.

43. Surveys of research on AIDS include Peter J. Fishinger, "Acquired Immune Deficiency Syndrome: The Causative Agent and the Evolving Perspective," *Current Problems in Cancer* 9(1): 1–39 (1985); John I. Gallin and Anthony S. Fauci, eds., *Acquired Immune Deficiency Syndrome (AIDS)*, Advances in Host Defense Mechanisms, vol. 5 (New York: Raven Press, 1985); Michael S. Gottlieb and Jerome E. Groopman, eds., *Acquired Immune Deficiency Syndrome*, Proceedings of a Shering Corporation–UCLA Symposium Held in Park City, Utah, February 5–10, 1984 (New York: Alan R. Liss, 1984). Initial articles on the discovery of the virus by French and American investigators are in *Science* 220: 868–71 (May 20, 1983); 224: 497–500; 500–503; 503–5; 506–8 (May 4, 1984); 607–10 (May 11, 1984).

44. Wyngaarden, "Nurturing the Scientific Enterprise," p. 160.

45. Judith P. Swazey and Karen Reeds, *Today's Medicine, Tomorrow's Science: Essays on Paths of Discovery in the Biomedical Sciences* (Washington, D.C.: U.S. Department of Health, Education & Welfare, DHEW Publication No. (NIH) 78-244), p. 116.

46. Wyngaarden, "Nurturing the Scientific Enterprise," p. 159.

47. For the most recent statement of this philosophy, see Wyngaarden, "Directions and Challenges," p. 274.

48. On the origin of Consensus Development Conferences see Donald S. Fredrickson, "The Purposes of the National Institutes of Health. I. On the Translation Gap," in "Speeches, Articles, and Selected Papers," 1: document 1 (July 1975).

49. Donald S. Fredrickson, "A History of Recombinant DNA Guidelines in the United States," in Joan Morgan and W. J. Whelan, eds., *Recombinant DNA and Genetic Experimentation* (Oxford and New York: Pergamon Press, 1979), pp. 151–56; also published in *Recombinant DNA Technical Bulletin* 2: 87–90 (1979).

50. Kenneth J. Cremer et al., "Vaccina Virus Recombinant Expressing

Herpes Simplex Virus Type 1 Glycoprotein D Prevents Latent Herpes in Mice," *Science* 228: 737–40 (May 10, 1985).

51. "Blood Oxygenator Membranes," in *Research Advances* (Washington, D.C.: Government Printing Office, 1975, DHEW Publication No. (NIH) 75-3), pp. 30–31.

52. J. E. Rall, "Epilogue," in Stetten and Carrigan, eds., *NIH: An Account of Research in Its Laboratories and Clinics*, pp. 527–28.

53. Shryock, *Development of Modern Medicine*, p. 457.

Index

References to illustrations are printed in italic type

The Johns Hopkins University Press

Inventing the NIH

This book was set in Century Old Style text and display type by EPS Group, from a design by Chris L. Smith. It was printed on 50-lb. Sebago Eggshell Cream Offset paper and bound in Holliston's Payko by BookCrafters.